HOMOEOPATHY
AND CHILDREN

By the same author:-

Homoeopathic Medicine

The Homoeopathic Treatment of Emotional Illness

A Woman's Guide to Homoeopathy

Understanding Homoeopathy

Talking About Homoeopathy

An Encyclopedia of Homoeopathy

The Principles, Art and Practice of Homoeopathy

Emotional Health

Personal Growth and Creativity

The Side-Effects Book

HOMOEOPATHY FOR BABIES AND CHILDREN

A Guide to Remedies for the Young Family

by

Dr Trevor Smith
MA, MB, Bchir, DPM, MFHom

INSIGHT

Insight Editions
Worthing, Sussex
England

WARNING

The contents of this volume are for general interest only and individual persons should always consult their medical adviser about a particular problem or before stopping or changing an existing treatment.

Insight Editions
Worthing
Sussex
England

Published by Insight Editions 1993

British Library Cataloguing in Publication Data

A catalogue record for this book is available
from the British Library.

ISBN 0-496670 15 3

Cover photograph by the author.

INTRODUCTION

Homoeopathy is a safe natural way of treating your baby or young child, using diluted natural extracts, usually of plant, or mineral origin. These provide a safe gentle stimulus to health.

Homoeopathy deals with the whole person, but what is most important, it deals with the psychological needs of the individual child. Its guiding principle is treating 'like by like', or choosing a remedy which in its original form was capable of causing symptoms similar to those the child may be experiencing in his present illness.

Homoeopathy supports the young mother who wants more initiative and more involvement in the treatment of the family. It provides an independent approach to the health problems of her child, providing a safe method which supports the subtle energies responsible for the resistance and health of the child.

Once the homoeopathic approach has been understood, the mother can approach the problems of the individual child with more confidence, which reassures the child.

Although most mothers have heard about homoeopathy, they are not usually well-informed by the health visitor or midwife about its value. It is understandable that the mother tends to be sceptical and cautious.

Being a mother can be worrying and many feel in a dilemma, trapped by the wish to treat their child with a natural method, but fearing their doctor will disapprove.

Many mothers are concerned about the long-term effects of repeated prescriptions upon the health of the child. Homoeopathy offers a safe alternative without causing side-effects. When a conventional drug is essential, it supports the its action without reducing its activity.

Any young mother can get into a panic when her angry, screaming baby has wind or colic and demands instant relief from discomfort. But she should try to keep a sense of humour and balance with her child all the time; enjoying playing, talking, holding and touching him. If the child is difficult, remember that there are no difficult children - only different children.

Each child develops his patterns of behaviour by learning from example. It is not so much what you say, but how you say it, that determines his understanding and responses. If you don't want your child to shout or swear, then don't shout or swear at the child. Don't hit the child if you don't want him to hit back at you.

Try to approach all pressure situations calmly, without the use of bribes, smacking, or physical threats. If you must punish, some form of temporary restriction is often more effective, but always explain your reasons and the aspect of behaviour you disagree with.

At all times respect the child as a person and an individual, even if you feel he has upset you or behaved badly. If he has been childish or immature, this is only to be expected from one who is only beginning to climb the ladder of social skills and graces.

7, Upper Harley Street
London NWI 4PS

SOME GENERAL ADVICE FOR PARENTS ON TAKING HOMOEOPATHIC REMEDIES.

The remedies recommended throughout the book should be purchased directly from a homoeopathic pharmacy or health shop. Always ensure that your remedies are from a reliable source and used in the 6c potency.

The potencies or strengths, come as small round pills or tablets, made of sucrose (or lactose). If you are sensitive to lactose, you should order your remedies directly from a homoeopathic pharmacy, requesting a sucrose or lactose-free pill base for the remedies. Because the medicine or homoeopathic dilution is applied directly to the surface of the pill, they should not be handled. They are best placed directly into the mouth from the lid of the container and sucked under the tongue. They should always be taken on a clean mouth, at least 30 minutes before or after food or drink (except water), orthodox medicines, vitamin or mineral supplements, and toothpaste.

Do not drink peppermint tea when taking homoeopathic remedies. Avoid coffee, tea and cocoa, because their high caffeine content may diminish the homoeopathic effect.

The medicines should be stored in a cool, dry, dark area, away from strong odours, especially camphor, oil of wintergreen, perfume, essential oils, after-shave and soap. In this way, their action will last indefinitely.

A bland diet is recommended, not eating to excess, or using strong spices. Alcohol should be avoided, and smoking should be reduced or stopped altogether during the period of treatment, especially for lung, heart, or circulatory problems.

Remedies should be taken for as long as any symptoms persist - and then stopped. If new symptoms arise during homoeopathic treatment, they should be watched carefully, especially if they have occurred in the past. The homoeopathic action may sometimes cause earlier symptoms to reappear. They are usually fleeting, but if persistent, they will require a new remedy.

Any increase (aggravation) of symptoms, after taking the remedy, is a positive sign, and indicates a response. It is usually short-lived, and does not undermine the overall sense of well-being. Do not continue taking a remedy once the symptoms have improved.

If your overall condition deteriorates after taking a homoeopathic remedy, stop taking the remedy and consult your homoeopathic doctor.

There are no side-effects or risks from homoeopathy. If you take a wrong remedy, or a whole box of the 6c pills, they will cause no harm. The remedies can be safely used during pregnancy, breast-feeding, or given to the youngest baby.

Homoeopathic remedies do not interact with orthodox medicines, or undermine their action. If you are given a course of antibiotics, it is best to stop homoeopathic remedies until you have ceased the antibiotics.

Some orthodox drugs, especially steroids, may reduce or neutralise the homoeopathic effect.

If parents are concerned about putting the very small homoeopathic pills into the baby's mouth, although this is not a risk, they can crush the pills, between two spoons to create a fine powder, which can then be put on the child's tongue.

Homoeopathy is not a treatment for acute or severe pain and orthodox treatment is recommended if this occurs. Homoeopathy acts at every age, the reaction varying with age, strength and the resistance or vital energy reserves of the patient. It acts very quickly in a child, or fit young person, but is slower in an elderly person, particularly if old, weak, or feeble.

It is often better initially, to give an orthodox treatment to an elderly person during the acute stage of an illness, using homoeopathy when they are recovering, or before they are in acute illness or weakness.

Homoeopathy is nevertheless helpful in the older age group - for stiffness, constipation, insomnia or anxiety. It does not cause confusion or agitation, which can be a severe problem when orthodox drugs are used.

ACCIDENT PRONENESS

This may be of physical or emotional origin. Where the problem has a physical causation, it is usually associated with problems of co-ordination from neurological damage. In some cases the cause is a precipitate birth with excessive pressures in the birth canal and anoxia. More rarely the causes are due to a metabolic disorder, or a genetic syndrome.

Homoeopathy can help where the underlying cause is physical, but it is often more supportive than curative, the child needing other specialised help and backup, especially where the problem is severe. Most common is accident proneness associated with an underlying emotional disorder of some kind. The child tends to be quick and precipitate in all things, always off balance and ready to dash off and do something which ends in disaster. Usually the child is trying to be helpful and is very willing to lend a hand, but inevitably whatever he does, it ends in a fall, cut, or bruise because he is off balance and does not pace himself or know how to slow down. The child's writing and reading, indeed his whole learning process, may be affected with this same tendency to dash forward into the next word, sentence or idea, before the present one has been properly taken in and understood. For this reason, he often loses confidence and attention, is always in trouble, and frequently compensates by drawing attention to himself by some other form of risky behaviour which again ends in disaster and is counterproductive. Because of this same tendency to rush ahead of himself, he tends to be old before his time, or pseudo-mature, typically associating with older children rather than his own peer group. The child may require some individual tuition to restore confidence.

Remedies to consider include :

Arnica
Useful where the problem follows a head injury or concussion. The child is bruised psychologically since that time, never fully recovered, poorly co-ordinated, woolly in thinking and slow in perception of time and space.

Helleborus
Helpful where the problem follows an accident or head-injury of some kind. Vagueness, concentration poor, impaired perceptual ability is typical, with sighing. There is slowing of all reactions.

Lycopodium
The child is quick and precipitate in thinking and movement, but timing and balance are poor. He is tilted forwards emotionally, as if always on starting blocks of life, too eager, clumsy and often in a wrong position. Anticipatory fear is a feature, the child anxious to please, needing reassurance in all things.

Kali carb
The child lacks the energy of Lycopodium. He tends to feel depressed or anxious lacking confidence, especially if on his own. Fearful about most things, tension and accident-prone.

ADENOID PROBLEMS

Adenoids are a thickening of the normal lymphoid tissue within the nasopharynx (part of the throat behind the soft palate, at the base of the nasal area), leading to almost constant blockage of the nose, and as a result, to mouth breathing.

This may cause a nasal speech and a constantly blocked nose, snoring, or recurrent infections, particularly of the throat, sinuses and nasal region. The infection may also involve the upper chest bronchial area, with frequent chesty colds.

If the enlarged adenoid tissue blocks the eustachian tube, joining the posterior part of the throat and the middle ear, it may lead to temporary deafness or recurrent middle ear infections (otitis media).

Because all lymphatic tissues acts as an important natural barrier to infection, for example - the tonsils, it is inadvisable to remove them surgically unless there is a very severe problem of obstruction.

Enlarged adenoids should not be removed routinely, or just because they are large. This is quite normal at this age, and they form an important part of the body's defence system.

Remedies to consider :

Antimonium crud The tongue has a white coating, the voice affected - croaky or weak.

Baryta carb The throat is red, painful and inflamed, the lymphatic glands of the neck tender and enlarged. Swallowing is painful.

Calcarea carb Lethargy and chill are characteristic. There is a sour taste in the mouth. Swallowing is painful.

Hepar sulph There is acute inflammation, with splinter-like pains, and thick yellow purulent mucus.

Phosphorus Useful for acute adenoid problems with weakness and a blood-stained discharge. All symptoms are better for cold drinks. Anxiety and tension are marked.

Psorinum There is a foul, dirty unpleasant throat discharge, the symptoms better for heat, worse for cold air.

Pulsatilla There is a variable greenish-yellow mucus catarrh, all symptoms aggravated by heat.

AGGRESSIVE BEHAVIOUR AND IRRITABILITY

This is common in all children at some time as simple naughtiness and it should be seen as normal and not made into a drama or treated in an over-punitive way that may damage the child. All children break the rules at times as an expression of their natural curiosity, instincts and need to find out the limits of their environment. In many ways, the child who is never naughty, is an unhealthy child. If repetitive, and there is a problem in a specific area, perhaps with a particular adult or child, it should be talked about.

There may be a problem of jealousy or resentment, which should be discussed, making the child feel more secure and cared about, and ensuring that he is given sufficient individual time and attention from both parents. If there is no obvious reason for the aggressive bouts, or there is a sudden change in the pattern of behaviour, the child should be seen by a paediatrician to establish that the problem is emotional and that there is not an underlying physical cause.

Changes in behaviour with aggressive outbursts sometimes occur after an accident involving a head injury with concussion. If childbirth has been precipitate, the head rushed through the birth canal, or subject to lack of oxygen at this time, there may have been subtle damage to the brain tissues which can in later life cause irritable aggressive behaviour. Other causes include incipient epilepsy, often with a history of fits in another close member of the family. In most cases however the cause is a psychological one and this needs exploration and time. Some individual counselling may also be required in addition to the remedies.

Remedies to consider:

Nux vomica Intense bouts of irritation occur in a short-fuse, tense personality. Spasms of tension and anger are associated with impatience.

Chamomilla There is restless sudden anger with a constant need for attention. Intolerant, spiteful and complaining behaviour. He is better for being held and cuddled, worse when put down.

Lilium tig There is a combination of irritable aggressive behaviour with anxiety and depression.

Tarentula hisp A remedy for destructive mood changes. The child tears clothes and sheets and is extremely irritability and restless.

ALLERGIC RHINITIS

This is one of the most common childhood problems, the nose blocked due to swelling of the mucosal lining and producing varying amounts of mucus. This may be watery, or frequently there is a thick yellow-green mucus production.

The child usually feels miserable, the nose constantly blocked or running, mucus dropping back onto the throat and waking him at night. Allergic causes vary, but are often specific for the individual child.

Some of the commonest are milk products, chocolate, cheese, pollen, especially rape seed and Timothy grass. Rhinitis is often caused by house-dust, due to the house-dust mite. Desensitization treatment may be used, but in the writer's experience, it is rarely really successful.

When rhinitis becomes persistent or a chronic and recurrent problem the child often becomes irritated or depressed. If this occurs, he should be give extra time, reassurance and encouragement and not be punished, or seen as just naughty.

The homoeopathic approach is to build up the resistance of the individual child and to use specific homoeopathic allergic remedies. These include grasses, house dust, cat or dog hair, or any specific irritant made into a remedy by the homoeopathic pharmacist.

Remedies to consider:

Kali bich There is usually a chronic persistent nasal catarrh in an overweight child who lacks energy. The discharge is thick, stringy, greenish mucus. Mouth breathing occurs because both nostrils are blocked. A post-nasal drip may cause a choking type of discomfort at night.

Kali Carb The child is apathetic, often overweight because of an excessive dairy food intake, with chronic thick yellow nasal catarrh. Symptoms are often worse in the early hours, the child waking with a cough or unable to breath because of nasal congestion. Restlessness with marked anxiety is often present.

ANXIETY

Children quickly become anxious because their security is often fragile in the early developmental years. But few parents realise how anxious a child can feel, particularly in any new or unfamiliar situation. Childhood fears are always magnified, causing tension, often terror, especially when the child has not been included in the preparations for any new or strange situation, such as a new school, another child or partner coming into the house, the break-up of a marriage or relationship. When a change of this order is not discussed openly with the child, he becomes anxious because his fantasy life takes over, sometimes to an extreme degree because of the type of fairy-tale imagery children conjure up. Unless balanced by reality information from the parents, often helped by an older sibling, the child's fantasy imagery can cause anxiety because it is confused with reality.

The most common manifestations of anxiety in the child are symptoms of insecurity - whining, demanding, sometimes fear of going to sleep, or turning the light off. Other common anxiety symptoms are increased thumb-sucking, or a recurrence of bed-wetting, sometimes skin problems such as eczema. In some children there may be diarrhoea or asthma.

Whenever there are anxiety problems, children should be encouraged to express their feelings and discuss them with their parents, encouraged to feel that their demands and insecurity are quite normal and appropriate. No child should be told or taught to bottle-up feelings, or to feel guilty about them.

Remedies to consider:

Aconitum   For acute anxiety problems where fear is marked.

Argentum nit   For the phobic very anxious child who is anxious about any new situation involving meeting others, or when he feels he will be on display. Phobic children are more anxious in a warm or over-heated room.

Gelsemium   Moderate anxiety problems are present, mainly of a dramatic type.

Lycopodium   Where the child is full of anticipatory terrors and fears. Worse in the afternoon or early evening, always clumsy and too quick off the mark.

Natrum mur   For the insecure child, never at ease in company, fearful of strangers and other children, tearful and often depressed.

Sulphur   Where the child is muddled and anxious, unrealistic in his approach to problems.

APPETITE INCREASE OR DECREASE.

The desire for food quite naturally varies with every child according to his physical and psychological health and the body constitution. Usually the healthy child has a good appetite,but it is not endless and it varies. A large framed active child will eat more than a child who is less active, more artistic or intellectual, and where the body frame is smaller.

Appetite also varies with the family and some families overindulge their children with food which creates unhealthy appetite patterns and a foundation for illness in adult life. The over-weight child is not healthy and may be linked to diabetes later in life, especially where the child was born heavy, continues to put on weight, or becomes fat and flabby.

The slim child is not unhealthy as long as he has a varied adequate diet which satisfies him. Let the child eat as much as he feels like and don't push food down him in the mistaken belief that the bigger the child the healthier he will become. High cholesterol levels in adults and an increased risk of heart disease is now known to be associated with faulty eating habits which begin in childhood.

The foundations of healthy adulthood should be encouraged by offering a diet that is low in fats, sugar and salt from the beginning, with the emphasis on a high intake of cereal fibre, fresh vegetables and fruit. If there is a diminished appetite, this is often psychological or due to infection, also when the child is incubating an infection. If it persists, consult your homoeopathic doctor for a medical opinion.

Remedies to consider:- for excess appetite :

Sulphur

The child is continuously hungry for any kind of food, especially fatty or fried foods, chips, crisps, or sweet foods. Indigestion is marked with a sour taste in the mouth, a dirty yellow tongue and windy stomach distention.

Ask your homoeopathic doctor to give the child a constitutional remedy.

Remedies to consider:- for appetite loss.

Baryta carb

For the weak child, slow to reach his growth milestones, always chilly, with problems of chronic nasal catarrh or recurrent adenoid or tonsillar infections.

Silicea

A useful remedy for the weak sickly child, often as a result of poor nutrition or following a bad reaction to immunisation. The child is thin and chilly, every injury tending to heal slowly or becomes infected. Vital resistance is low. These children usually lack confidence and drive.

Tuberculinum

For the thin pale often energetic child with no appetite. He usually has a recurrent dry cough and a tendency to chest weakness.

ASTHMA

Shortness of breath and wheezing attacks of allergic origin sometimes occur in the young child of a few months. Often the child has suffered from recurrent coughs and colds since birth. These may eventually develop into bronchitis with breathing difficulties.

Later, the typical asthma problem of not getting enough air into the lungs (because the bronchial tubes are in spasm) and high-pitched musical sounds on breathing-out tend to occur.

Often the mother or father is also affected with a similar asthmatic problem, or another member of the family. However a family asthmatic link does not always occur. Symptoms are often worse in the early hours as the temperature drops, or in cold damp conditions.

It is essential that the child is under medical supervision as soon as the condition is diagnosed.

Many asthmatic children are sensitive, often because of a nervous temperament. It is important to encourage them to express any fears or anxieties they have in order to maximise dialogue and discussion within the family, and to have contacts with other children. They should not be over-protected, but at the same time not exposed to family tensions and feuds at an impressionable age which is likely to create fear or anxiety. Parents should always give psychological support and a sense of security to the child whenever he becomes distressed by asthmatic symptoms.

Remedies to consider:

Ipecacuanha   For childhood asthma with copious sputum and a 'moist ' chest with loud coughing and often nausea or vomiting.

Gelsemium   For mild asthmatic problems, often where every cold goes onto the chest and causes spasm and a tendency to breathing difficulties. Anxiety is commonly associated.

Kali carb   For the overweight child who lacks energy and is constantly complaining of being tired. Recurrent nasal and throat catarrhal problems are a feature. He often lacks confidence and is irritable, moody and depressed.

Phosphorus   For more severe asthmatic problems, usually in a bright outgoing child. The attacks often occur at night, on lying down and because the child feels hot and thirsty.

Sambucus niger   For asthmatic problems usually occurring in the early hours, about midnight. The child starts to cough and this then leads onto asthmatic spasm and shortness of breath.

BAD BREATH

This may be associated with a dental problem, especially where there is a food trap which allows decaying food to accumulate. Equally it may be linked to a digestive problem, often constipation, the whole of the intestine sluggish, causing fermentation and distention of the stomach area .

Other common causes are:- infection of the throat, tonsil, sinuses, or pharynx (back of the throat). Such infections may become recurrent and are best dealt with by increasing the overall health of the child by a well-balanced diet also regular exercise and giving the appropriate homoeopathic remedy.

Attention must be paid to the diet, ensuring that it is not too high in sugars and yeast-containing foods such as yogurt, which may encourage fermentation.

If a dental food trap is present, it should be corrected, and whenever there is a problem of breath odour, an early dental check for loss of a filling or dental decay is recommended.

The bowel should always be kept healthy, encouraging natural elimination without the use of laxatives, helped by a high fibre diet; for example one containing bran or a high residue content, as occurs with most fresh vegetables.

Remedies to consider:

Carbo veg An excellent remedy where there is associated acidity, heartburn and indigestion, the child drowsy and fearful, the tongue coated white or yellow.

Kali phos Anxiety and exhaustion are usually present when this remedy is indicated.The breath is putrid and foul, the tongue coated and slimy, as the associated diarrhoea, the stomach uncomfortable with colicky pains. The child is always worse for stress or excitement.

Sulphur The breath is putrid and unpleasant smelling, associated with stomach distention, foul eructations of gas from the mouth and rectum. The tongue is dirty looking. Morning diarrhoea with a foul-smelling watery stool is a common problem.

BED COVERINGS

These should always be light and comfortable so that the child is not too hot or sweats during the night.

It is particularly important for the young baby to be only lightly covered, preferably with a brushed cotton sheet. The baby should never be over-dressed, either at night or during the day, with a free flow of air around the young body.

Temperature control is poor during the early weeks, and the young child can easily over-heat, causing strain on the heart.

Cot deaths are now believed to be linked to hyperthermia and overheating the child. To help reduce the incidence, it is important never to let the young baby sleep on its tummy, but only on its side or back.

A duvet should not be used until the child is over one year of age. Parents should keep the child warm, but not excessively so.

If in spite of light bed-clothing the child is still too hot, the head or neck area wet with perspiration, then homoeopathy should be considered.

Remedies to consider:

Argentum nit For the fearful restless child who is intolerant of heat. There is usually an associated indigestion problem, with a gassy painful upper stomach distention or discomfort, also wind and belching.

Belladonna The child is hot, red, sweating, anxious and restless, with a raised pulse rate.

Calcarea carb The child is flabby and often overweight, usually chilly with a tendency to profuse sweating of the head. Typically he is slow to reach his expected milestones and fearful.

Pulsatilla For the rather placid child who is always too hot, tearful and emotional, pulling back the covers as too warm and then quickly feeling cold.

Sulphur Useful for the child who is always too hot, sweaty, with a tendency to be overweight. Indigestion problems occur with a foul-smelling stool, often morning diarrhoea. Lethargy and lack of concentration is characteristic, also dislike of washing.

BED WETTING

A common problem for the emotionally immature or sensitive child. It should be treated as quite normal until the age of three because bladder maturity varies enormously from one child to another. After that age it should be considered as a possible sign of emotional insecurity. In some children there is a fear of growing up and facing up to being more independent.

In many cases the problem exists because the mother is unconsciously clinging to the child, encouraging dependency, sometimes anxiety in the child, because the mother is not sure how she will cope as the child matures. As long as the child is immature and dependant, this can reassure a mother who lacks confidence. It is always important to know if the insecurity lies within the mother or the child.

In every child, where bed wetting is a problem, it should be dealt with openly, with a sympathetic non-punitive approach. The child should not drink too much late at night or watch television late in the evening. Often the child sleeps too deeply and fails to wake when the bladder is full. Lifting the child at night may be considered by the parents, as a stepping-stone to acquiring bladder-control skills and dryness at night, provided it does not cause the child sleep problems.

The family should look at possible emotional causes for the problem:- sometimes insecurity after the arrival of a new baby, or an illness within the family. There is often a family history of at least one of the parents acquiring bladder control late in their childhood.

Remedies to consider :

Baryta carb   For bed-wetting problems where there is immaturity without the anticipatory anxiety, eagerness, and pseudo-maturity of the Lycopodium character. The child is usually slow developing, held back, and often shy and retiring.

Equisetum   A useful secondary remedy for bladder weakness and incontinence. The bladder area is often uncomfortable and feels full or painful.

Lycopodium   For the anxious immature child who lacks confidence and tends always to cross his bridges before he reaches them. He has frequent difficulties in relaxing or getting off to sleep and then sleeps too deeply and does not wake up when his bladder is full. Often he drinks too much because he is thirsty from eating too many sweet snacks during the day.

BITES

These are usually caused by a domestic animal, e.g. dog or cat, at other times by animals in captivity - monkeys or other caged animals with or without provocation. Human bites also occur - either accidental or deliberate. They are common is young children and where there is damage to the skin or underlying tissues, these should be treated in the same way as any other bite.

Most bites are from small domestic animals and usually there is a graze or scratch. But small children are also attacked by larger aggressive breeds of dog, sometimes a family pet and for no apparent reason, the dog always previously docile. If a child is bitten when on holiday abroad, an anti-rabies inoculation is usually recommended. Your doctor or local casualty officer will arrange this for you.

Children, particularly those without pets of their own, should be taught not to approach strange dogs, especially large dogs and not to tease or provoke them. They should not however be frightened, when the risks and dangers are explained to them. If a child has been bitten, it is important that the parents give psychological support after the injury, to minimise fear and anxiety reactions within the child and to rebuild his confidence.

After a small bite, clean the area carefully with water, and apply Calendula cream, covering the wound with a clean dressing. Use Rescue Remedy or Aconitum to reduce a severe panic or anxiety reaction. If there is persistent bleeding from the wound, apply firm pressure. If the wound is large, take the child to the casualty department of your local hospital.

Remedies to consider:

Aconitum   For severe acutely distressing bites, often associated with fear or anxiety.The skin is usually red and swollen, hot, burning and painful.

Apis   For red, irritating painful swollen areas of skin, the child restless and anxious without thirst.

Arnica   Indicated where there is restlessness with anxiety, marked redness or bluish swelling of the area and a painful bruised sensation.

Ledum   In marked contrast to Aconitum, where this remedy is indicated, the area feels chilled and cold. But paradoxically the wound is also improved by a cold application and worse for any form of heat.

BLISTERS

These are often infective in origin, associated with one of the acute childhood infections, such as chicken-pox. If localised to one area, perhaps the heel or toe, they are usually due to friction from a prolonged walk, an ill-fitting unsuitable shoe, or faulty posture, when walking or running.

When there is a small crop of blisters which come and go, usually with tenderness and irritation; on the genital, thigh or buttock area, these may be caused by a herpes viral infection. They are infective and may be passed to other members of the family. Always discuss a problem of recurrent small blisters on the buttock or genital area with your doctor.

Most cases of genital herpes occur in adults and the majority of blisters that children experience, are due to a friction burn, the blister acting as a protective cushion to stop further damage.

Remedies to consider:

Apis The area is red swollen and painful with stinging sensitivity.

Natrum mur The skin is tender, with fluid retention in the area affected. There is anxiety with restlessness, the child better for fresh air.

Rhus tox For itchy redness with small blisters or pimples.

Varicellinum There are multiple tender blisters, which may discharge a clear fluid.

BOILS

These are a painful localised reaction to infection with redness, swelling, inflammation and pus formation. They are common in diabetes because of the high blood sugar levels, due to pancreatic malfunctioning, which encourages bacterial growth in the skin. But they also occur where there is a high intake of sugars in the diet, causing a similar condition to diabetes.

When boils are a problem, it is important to reduce the child's dietary intake of sugar and confectionary, including sugar taken as honey or fructose, also fruit sugars.

Recurrent boils are best treated by assessing the underlying cause and correcting this. Urinary and blood sugar levels should be carefully monitored in all diabetics and children with an excessive dietary sugar intake.

No child should be allowed to become overweight, and regular exercise as well as diet are helpful to keep weight to optimum levels for height and age.

Encourage the child to wash carefully after coming in from play, before eating and after a bowel action. From an early age, he should be aware of the importance of commonsense hygiene measures, as long as these are not exaggerated or over-emphasised.

Remedies to consider:

Antimonium crud   For severe burning itchy discharging localised infections. These are usually worse for heat, cold, or wet applications.

Apis   For recurrent boil problems, the skin red and tender. Irritable restlessness with anxiety.

Pulsatilla   For recurrent boils which come and go, often associated with a high carbohydrate intake. There are variations of mood with tearfulness. All symptoms are worse for heat of any kind.

Sulphur   For chronic boils, the skin dirty-looking and often infected. Acne or eczema may also be present.

BREATH HOLDING

This is common in nervous or tense children, where it may become a frightening problem, although it is not usually dangerous. The child or baby, holds its breath, and may go blue in the face to the point of fainting, and then breathes normally again.

The problem may tend to keep occurring as 'attacks' of breath holding, particularly when the child has been over-excited or in a tantrum. In some cases there is no known cause, and an emotional factor is not apparent, the child otherwise normal and calm.

Parents should always consider that there may be an underlying psychological element which is causing some tension and anxiety, and give the child the time and opportunity to express any fears or anxieties which may be worrying him.

If severe and repetitive, a paediatric specialist opinion should be sought to exclude the possibility of epilepsy.

Remedies to consider:

Natrum mur   A remedy where anxiety, tearfulness, tension and fear are marked features. Strangers are felt to be a threat because of the underlying insecurity. The child is usually worse for consolation, holding and reassurance; often preferring to be alone.

Nux vomica   Where there is irritability, the attacks coming in spasms, often provoked by temper tantrums or an emotional crisis. The problems tend to recur, usually provoked by emotion or frustration.

The child's constitutional remedy is often required, usually prescribed by your homoeopathic doctor.

BRONCHITIS

Infection of the bronchial passages may be acute and suddenly involve the chest of a previously healthy child, or follow an acute throat inflammation. The cause is either viral or bacterial, the latter more likely to be associated with a high temperature. In some children there is no apparent reason for the infection, or it may follow a chill, or the child may have always had a weak chest, perhaps a history of previous attacks.

A child who is weak, perhaps convalescent after an operation, living in a polluted, dusty, or damp environment is particularly prone to develop bronchitis. Children living near to main roads with a high volume of traffic and consequent air pollution, are particularly at risk.

Bronchitis is frequently the result of secondary smoking, and may become chronic. This is the reason why the mother should not smoke during pregnancy.

Neither parent should smoke in the home where a child is present, because of the risks of lung infection.

All children should have fresh air, good basic fresh food, regular exercise, their body weight kept to optimum levels, but not in excess.

The bonny fat baby or child should be positively discouraged.

Remedies to consider:

Bryonia
For recurrent chest problems with a dry irritating cough, tearing pains, worse for movement and better for rest. There is breathlessness on effort, the chest symptoms worse for heat.

Ipecacuanha
Nausea or vomiting occurs with breathlessness and a persistent noisy bubbling cough.

Natrum sulph
A remedy for severe recurrent bronchitis, with breathlessness on effort and all symptoms aggravated by cold or damp.

Lycopodium
A useful remedy used for right-sided chest problems, the symptoms worse in the early evening and aggravated by heat.

Phosphorus
For severe bronchitis with shortness of breath, aggravated by fear and anxiety. The child is thin weak and pale, craving cold drinks.

BRUISES

Bruises are usually due to a fall or blow damaging the delicate skin tissues. There is bleeding from fine blood vessels with haemorrhage into the surrounding area causing the typical blue discolouration.

Swelling is due to fluid retention in the area affected and there is also tenderness. Bruises are sometimes spontaneous, when the child has a fine skin and a tendency to bleeding.

The cause may be due to the type of skin, and delicate vessels which break and haemorrhage easily, or more serious reasons including genetic diseases such as Haemophilia.

Sometimes bruising occurs as a reaction to a prescribed drug which interferes with the normal blood clotting time, so that bleeding into tissues occurs at the slightest knock or trauma. On rare occasions, there is a toxic cause for the bruising, as during severe measles, or scarlet fever.

Reassurance from the parents, is important following the incident. A cold compress helps to reduce swelling and bruising then applying a soothing and healing homoeopathic cream of one of the recommended remedies to the bruised area. Also give the remedies by mouth, and continue until the condition has fully healed.

Remedies to consider:

Apis   There is redness and swelling with local heat and restlessness. Lack of thirst is a feature.

Arnica   For painful swollen inflamed areas, following a fall. Most symptoms are improved by a cold application.

Bellis perennis   An excellent remedy after Arnica for bruised swollen tissue injuries with nerve irritation or damage, from a fall or sprain. The area is sore and painful. Intolerance of cold applications is a feature, also feeling worse for local heat, but better for local strapping and support.

Ledum   The bruised discoloured area feels cold and chilled, but paradoxically is better for a cold compress and worse for heat.

Rhus tox   There is a painful sprained or bruised area, better for heat and aggravated by cold or damp.

CAR SICKNESS

This is a very common problem, especially for sensitive children due to a combination of an excitable temperament and the movements of the car, on the internal balance organs of the inner ear. It is always aggravated by reading in the car, or any concentrated attention to close-up detail when travelling.

Relaxing the child before any journey and preparing the child emotionally for the trip well in advance, with attention to any obvious anxiety areas, helps lessen the problem and also prevents the build-up of too much emotion. If the parents remain calm, this also tends to relax the child.

Always open windows when travelling by car and give the child plenty of fresh air. It is best not to allow the child to read in the car, as this may increase any feelings of nausea. Avoid heavy meals before leaving on a long journey, and allow frequent rest stops for a short break and a walk about. In this way the child can be kept more relaxed and at ease during the journey.

Remedies to consider:

Cocculus	For travel sickness with profuse salivation, always worse for the smell of food or any strong odours and relieved by lying down.

Nux vomica	There are usually colicky pains associated with the nausea. Irritation, peevish ill-temper and anger also occurs. Constipation is a feature.

Petroleum	A useful remedy for severe nausea and giddiness, followed by hunger. All the symptoms are improved by eating.

Pulsatilla	There are variable symptoms, usually from emotional causes, with tears and intolerance of any form of heat.

CHICKENPOX

Chickenpox or Varicella is one of the commonest acute infective illness of childhood. Most children catch the infection at some time, usually before puberty, with subsequent lifetime immunity. The incubation period is approximately 18 to 21 days. Before the rash develops, the child is usually vaguely unwell, with less interest in food and playing, or lethargic and whining, lacking in normal energy.

The typical rash covers the body with dark red pimples, in various phases of development, including blister-like vesicles, which contain a clear fluid, small ulcer-like scabs, or raw red areas. This phase of the illness usually lasts over four to five days, At this time a young child often feels quite well, better once the rash has developed, although an older child who develops a high temperature may feel unwell and be completely lethargic and often restless. At the time of the rash, the child is highly infectious, and should be kept away from young babies, the elderly and any child who is convalescent or weak from any cause. The finger nails should be kept very short.

Complications are rare and most children recover fully without further problems, the course of the illness lasting about 2 weeks. At times the infection takes a more acute and severe form, with a high temperature, a severe diffuse rash, with a secondary bacterial infection, leading to scarring. Rarely it takes a neurological course and the viral infection involves the brain with meningitis or encephalitis. Apply calamine lotion, also Calendula or Rhus tox cream, to the most irritating areas of the rash.

Remedies to consider :

Antimonium crud   This remedy is helpful during the early phase of an irritating rash with various phases of pimples, blisters and scab formation.

Natrum mur   The skin is greasy and infected, the child pale, anxious and tearful.

Psorinum   There is the typical rash, the child covered with perspiration, weak and debilitated. All symptoms are aggravated by cold or a draught and better for heat.

Rhus tox   There is an itchy rash with restlessness and amelioration by heat.

Sulphur   The child is hot, ill-tempered and restless, yet constantly hungry. The skin looks dirty and has a varied rash, which is often discharging. Early morning diarrhoea is common.

Varicellinum   The specific vaccine-equivalent homoeopathic nosode for the condition and often indicated for all but very mild cases to help prevent the disease where infection is undesirable.

CIRCUMCISION

Circumcision is widely practised throughout the world for medical, religious, racial, and primitive tribal reasons. But it should only ever be carried out on strictly medical grounds, as it is a surgical procedure and potentially a trauma and risk for the child.

Where there is narrowing of the external meatus, with obstruction and ballooning of the prepuce, circumcision is necessary, and it is best done by a paediatric surgeon in a specialised unit.

Any intervention of a painful and surgical nature is best avoided unless strictly necessary, the child allowed to enter into life with minimal trauma. Every anaesthetic or operation carries a slight risk, particularly from haemorrhage after the operation.

Circumcision does not make the male penis cleaner or healthier, and it does not prevent cancer occurring in the female partner at a later stage. It may however affect later personality development because it is a painful trauma to the young male at a critical and early stage in his psychological development.

Remedies to consider:

Aconitum   When the child has not reacted well to the operation, is fearful and in a state of psychological shock.

Arnica   This is useful both before and after the operation.

Phosphorus   A remedy that may be useful where the child is nervous and restless, with a tendency for post-operative bleeding to occur.

Staphysagria   For the child who complains of post-operative stitch-like discomfort or pain, the child feeling irritable or resentful.

COLD SORES

These are caused by infection with the oral (mouth) herpes virus, and are common at any age, but particularly at a time when the child is tired and run-down, or convalescent.

A cold sore often complicates a viral common cold, or when the child is low following a spate of recurrent throat or sinus infections.

They are highly infective to the young baby and any child with a cold sore should be kept well away and all contacts avoided, until the sore has dried up. They may last for several weeks and are common on the upper or lower lip.

A cold sore carries no risk and they eventually clear-up spontaneously. They tend however to re-occur whenever the child is in a low, anxious, or fatigued state of mind, as at the end of term or sometimes just before an examination.

Remedies to consider:

Calcarea carb For the chilly sluggish overweight child who has a low vitality and is susceptible to every infection in the family. He sweats on the face and head at night. Nervous agitation is also present.

Causticum For the pale weak child, slow to reach his developmental milestones, the lip raw, burning and very sore. Useful for recurrent cold sores.

Kali carb For cold sores of the upper lip, improved by local heat, the child waking at 4-5.00am thirsty for a drink and because of discomfort. Lack of energy, anxiety and a tendency to be overweight is also characteristic.

Natrum mur For cold sores of the lower lip, associated with dryness or cracking of the area, weakness and fatigue.

Nitric acid For painful cold sores with sharp or burning splinter-like pains.

Pulsatilla A cold sore is usually present in the centre of the lower lip, all symptoms worse for heat and improved in the fresh air.

COLDS

The common cold, of viral origin can occur at any age. It is particularly prevalent in children because of the infectious nature of the illness and the amount of social contact that children have with each other.

In the vast majority of cases, the common cold involves the nose and throat, (sometimes the sinuses with inflammation), causing a watery or thick discharge of mucous from the nasal passages, often with blockage of one or other nostril.

The nasal discharge may be yellow or green, the skin around the nose and lips raw and sore. A dry cough is also common and often a headache, with aching pains throughout the body.

In acute forms, the ears become involved leading to acute inner ear infection (otitis media).There is often a slight temperature, although it may be over 100F(39C) if there is severe infection of the ears or an acute throat complication. Where this happens, the lymph nodes of the neck become enlarged and tender, often in one particular area, as they drain and try to halt the spread of the infection.

Remedies to consider:

Aconitum For very acute colds with shivering and pains in the throat or limbs. There is marked anxiety and restlessness.

Arsenicum The child has an acute chesty cold with exhaustion.

Influenzinum For typical flu-like colds with a high temperature, exhaustion, limb pains, diarrhoea or constipation.

Kali bich A remedy for colds with mainly nasal catarrh and exhaustion.

Kali carb Weakness and exhaustion is marked, usually with a throat infection and painful neck glands. Anxiety is often a feature.

Nux vomica For acute colds with spasms of abdominal pain, constipation and irritability.

Pulsatilla There is variable nasal or throat congestion, with greenish- yellow catarrh and sinus congestion. All symptoms are worse from heat.

Pyrogen Indicated for shivering attacks, a high fever, restlessness and delirium.

COLIC

There is a painful condition of griping pains which double-up the child or baby because of the intensity of the spasms. They are usually associated with indigestion and wind, often from rapid eating or too much food (either solids or at the breast).

Usually colic occurs because of an excessive fluid intake, which is taken too quickly. When this occurs in a young baby it is important to hold him up and to 'wind' the child during feeding, especially if he is taking too much milk together with a lot of swallowed air, swelling the intestine and causing colicky pains.

Good bottle and breast feeding technique is important in reducing the possibility of colic in a baby. If in doubt about correct feeding techniques, or colic is persistent or severe, advice should be obtained from your health visitor or midwife.

In an older child, colic may be intestinal in origin, associated with a dietary indiscretion of some kind, such as rushing meals, or not allowing the process of digestion to occur at a reasonable pace.

Where unripe food is eaten, or it has been polluted in some way, or there is an allergic reaction, colic is part of the body's natural process of elimination. Intestinal colic is usually associated with diarrhoea.

Remedies to consider:

Aconitum   For acute colicky conditions, with restlessness, extreme panic or fear. There is often a raised temperature.

Magnesium phos   For colicky pains which are relieved by doubling over, or by applying local heat to the area.

Nux vomica   For colicky conditions with spasm, constipation and irritability.

COMFORTERS

These are familiar objects - often pieces of cloth or a toy - which the child clings to as a source of reassurance. The object itself is not important, but it is usually something warm, soft, and cuddly.

The importance of comforters is that they reassure the child and are something he can control. In most children this is no more than a passing phase and attachment.

Where it is becomes a persistent habit, or interferes with learning or social relationships, it may need some counselling and explorative help, to look at the sources of any obvious anxiety problems.

Comforters are important temporary or transitional psychological objects, reassuring to the dependent child, and often a substitute for any anticipated loss of the mother.

Parents should never attempt to force a comforter from the child.

Remedies to consider:

Chamomilla   There is clinging anxiety with irritability, often associated with teething problems.

Lycopodium   There are marked anticipatory fears, reluctance to go anywhere new or to meet strangers. Indigestion problems are common with wind and flatulence and usually of nervous origin.

Pulsatilla   The child is clinging, lacks confidence, is fearful of the dark and shy of strangers. He is tearful at the slightest change.

Silicea   For the child who is thin, chilly, and who has sweaty feet. He tends to back away from any involvements because of lack of confidence.

CONFIDENCE LOSS

Confidence is essential for every child. It is largely the responsibility of the mother, but both parents are closely involved. Confidence or security in the self is usually present at birth, although it may be undermined by a traumatic delivery. It is essential for a child to sense that his mother is confident in herself, in her handling of the child and in their relationship. Although confidence is natural in most children from the start, it can be damaged by others, including the parents, by a jealous sibling, or a grandparent, in some cases by other children. The mother needs to keep an eye on the child's natural emergence as an individual, encouraging the child to explore and to make mistakes as part of natural growth and learning. It is important to avoid imposing set values, standards of behaviour, tidiness, or any patterns which make the child feel guilty or inadequate. The mother should try to remain calm as the child explores. She should not allow any of her own fears of new situations to frighten the child, taking reasonable safety precautions, without panic or excess emotion whenever the child does something new or different. Every child needs a variety of experiences with people and situations so that he can learn and relate to them, building experience and identifications for later life. A mother should ensure that as her child becomes more adventurous, he is not censored unnecessarily, or punished for natural curiosity and explorative behaviour. Never frighten, intimidate or threaten a child. Allow him to build courage as he discovers his environment, other people and other children. Give him maximum time to play with a variety of simple toys and enjoy his emerging spontaneity, identity and confidence.

Remedies to consider:

Aconitum

Where there is acute fear with restlessness and panic. There may be remoteness from others because of anxiety. The motivations of others and their communications are easily confused or misinterpreted.

Lycopodium

For the immature child who panics easily, never really at ease with others, although he gives the impression of being old for his years. The major problem is wanting to make haste too quickly so that he is psychologically off-balance and tilted into the future by anticipatory anxieties.

Natrum mur

For the child who is tearful and shuns others, in this way cutting down on some essential life experiences. Confidence is weak because of fears and anxiety, based on fantasies of what might happen, or a conviction of failure.

CONGESTION (NASAL)

A common problem for every young child and usually symptomatic of a mild infection in the nasal passages. It is occasionally associated with sinus problems or polyps, in some cases a deviated nasal septum.

If the septum is severely deviated, causing narrowing of one nasal passage, it may be advisable to have a paediatric surgical opinion with a view to re-aligning the nose.

When multiple and causing a blockage, nasal polyps may also have to be removed surgically, but recurrent operations are not recommended. If there is no evidence of narrowing due to an óbstructive cause, then every attempt should be made to increase the natural vitality and resistance of the child. This is best achieved using homoeopathy and ensuring a varied diet with plenty of fresh vegetables and fruit, including some eaten raw each day, also adequate exercise and fresh air.

If there is a stress or anxiety problem,it should be dealt with as soon as it is noticed and not left to fester where it may aggravate the congestion or other health problems. In some children, the problem is allergic and seasonal, for example hay-fever.

Remedies to consider:

Kali bich   The nose is blocked most of the time, also the sinuses. The area is tender to the point of pain with a thick yellow-green discharge. The area is dry and the sense of smell is often reduced or lost.

Pulsatilla   For variable nasal congestion with a yellow-greenish discharge; worse for heat; aggravated by a high intake of sugars and carbohydrates. All symptoms are worse for heat. The child is often tearful.

Sulphur   For chronic nasal catarrh that never seems to clear, worse for water or swimming. The child is often feeling too hot and always hungry. There is a foul-smelling and dirty-looking nasal discharge. Nose bleeds and adenoid problems are other common symptoms.

CONSTIPATION

This is usually the result of a faulty diet coupled with lack of proper bowel training of the child and often aggravated by the early use of laxatives. Where an adequate amount of vegetable and cereal fibre is provided in the diet, the roughage is usually perfectly adequate to stimulate a bowel movement each day. When this has been a problem in the past and laxatives have been resorted to, however natural, they tend to make for a lazy bowel and for chronic problems which may set the pattern for similar adult problems.

The child should be encouraged to evacuate at a regular time each day, but it should not be made a fetish or an anxiety situation, a win-or-lose psychological game which is harmful for the child and creates tensions and insecurities. If the child does not have a natural bowel movement at a particular time, then encourage him to have one at any other time of the day when he feels the urge to empty the bowel.

If he is constipated, don't worry or make an issue out of it. Let the child remain so and try the next morning or whenever you sense would be the natural time for the child to have an evacuation. Should the child go for several days without an evacuation, remain calm and relaxed, giving the child some extra bran, (about a teaspoonful a day is plenty). Figs or prunes soaked overnight are a useful stimulus to bowel evacuation. Always ensure that he is having plenty of fresh vegetables and fruit and an adequate intake of fluids. If he sweats a lot, give additional fluids especially when the climate is warm and humid. Avoid aluminium pans for food preparation, as these may be a causative factor.

Remedies to consider:

Alumina

For severe problems of constipation associated with itching in the area around the anus. Even after a hard mass of small round pellet-like stools are eventually passed with the greatest difficulty, the bowels still feel full.

Bryonia

For severe constipation problems, the child passing a large dry stool which is painful. The bowel problems are always worse for heat, hot drinks or a hot bath and for exercise.

Nux vomica

The desire to empty the bowel is weak or absent, the stool small and only partly evacuated. The constipation is painful and associated with irritability.

Opium

Where there is pain in the rectal and anal area from the hard mass of faeces present, but with an absence of any desire to evacuate. The stools which are eventually passed are dark or black. This is an important remedy for very obstinate constipation problems of the child.

CONVULSIONS

A febrile convulsion only occur when a young child has a raised temperature, particularly during an acute infective illness, such as measles or chickenpox, or sometimes during the course of an ear or throat infection.

Febrile convulsions should not be confused with, or thought of as a real convulsion, or epileptic fit. With epilepsy, the fit occurs without a raised temperature being present. The symptoms may be very brief, lasting a few seconds or over a period of a minute or two, the child's eyes rolling upwards into his head, with a brief spasmodic movement, or sometimes the child becomes remote and absent. Inform your doctor, as soon as the fit has passed and the child is back to normal.

If fits become continuous, recurring within a short period of time, or lasting over a period of a few minutes, telephone your doctor urgently or the emergency ambulance service to have the child admitted to hospital.

A history of epileptic fits may be a contra-indication to Whooping Cough vaccination because of a heightened risks of brain damage. In a sensitive child, fits may be a reaction to a prescribed drug he is taking, or because a drug has been stopped suddenly.

Any form of fit, either a very minor turn or a full-blown epileptic attack with biting of the tongue, loss of urinary control and loss of consciousness, should be discussed with your doctor. If there are other members of the family with this type of problem, discuss this too.

Remedies to consider:

Phosphorus   For the over-sensitive fidgety child who is restless, the fits often caused by too much excitement or anxiety.

Nux vomica   A remedy for the over-sensitive child with feelings which are too intense. He has poor controls and a short fuse temperament.

Helleborus   For fits following a head injury or trauma, including a long or precipitate birth. The child may be slow or overweight. All symptoms are worse in the late afternoon and early evening. Vomiting may also occur.

COUGH

This is a reflex action to clear the bronchial tubes of any irritant or foreign body. Usually the irritant is mucus from the throat, the result of smoking, a foreign body, piece of food, or a small insect.

In most cases it is associated with an upper bronchial tube infection, producing a lot of mucus which irritates the lung and causes the cough reflex to be constantly re-enacted.The remedies indicated depends upon the type of cough and whether it is productive.

Excessive coughing during the day or night in a young child who otherwise appears perfectly well, may indicate an allergic reaction, or a form of asthma.

A recurrent short cough may be stress-related and in a nervous child, the first sign of underlying nervousness and insecurity. If the cause is psychological, it is usually obvious to the family as it is triggered by an actual or anticipated emotional situation.

It is possible to take the homoeopathic remedies as a linctus, for example Bryonia, and this is often very useful for a young baby with a dry tickling cough who refuses the remedies in their usual pill form.

Remedies to consider:

Bryonia   For a dry cough, with a clear or white sputum.

Ipecacuanha   When the cough is moist with a large quantity of loose watery sputum.

Pulsatilla   The cough is moist and variable, with a greenish or thick catarrhal yellow sputum.

Phosphorus   For chesty coughs with shortness of breath and wheezing, often at night after lying down or when the bedroom temperature drops. The sputum may be blood-stained.

CRADLE CAP

This is a crusty seborrhoeic eruption on the scalp of the young baby. It is light brown in colour, and usually occurs at about the second or third week, lasting for three to four weeks.

In most cases it is perfectly harmless and of minor importance, affecting only a small area of the scalp. The area affected is often dry and flaking, giving the appearance that the baby has dandruff.

In a few cases, cradle cap becomes progressively more severe, spreading to involve a larger scalp area, and becoming thicker. This may become persistent, and if not treated and removed, it can last for months, even years, giving the child an unattractive appearance. The exact cause of cradle cap is unknown, but it is thought to be a type of eczema.

Shampoo the area twice weekly, using a gentle natural baby shampoo, and taking care not to irritate the baby's face or eyes. If it does persist, then homoeopathy is helpful, without putting the baby at risk.

Remedies to consider:

Calendula   This is helpful, and encourages healing. It is best used as a cream applied to the scalp in the morning and at night.

Rhus tox   For itchy dry eruptions on the head and scalp, worse for cold and draughts and better for warmth.

Sulphur   The eruptions are thick and grey-looking, often moist or slimy, aggravated by heat or water. Most of the irritation is worse on waking.

CROUP

Laryngeal spasm of the baby or young child, causes the characteristic croupy sound, as air is sucked through the narrowed larynx. It is almost always due to an infection, more rarely caused by an allergy.

If the croup becomes severe, the mother should remain confident and calm, in order to give the child confidence. Taking the child into a room moistened with steam, or a humid bathroom, will help him to breathe more easily.

Should the child remain distressed or seems to be worsening, or if he develops a high temperature, becoming short of breath, you should immediately contact your general practitioner. The doctor will then decide if the child needs to be admitted into hospital during the crisis, and cared for in a paediatric unit.

Croup is often more frightening for the mother than dangerous and it usually responds well to homoeopathy.

Remedies to consider:

Causticum   For croup with weakness or paralysis of the vocal chords, the child weak and restless. All symptoms are better for a moist atmosphere, as with steam inhalations and aggravated by draughts, or cold dry air.

Diphtherinum   For very severe attacks of croup, with weakness and collapse.

Nux vom   For spasmodic croup, worse in the morning. The throat is tight and irritable. All symptoms are worse for contact with dry cold air.

Sambucus   The croup is worse at night, the child hot and covered with sweat. His face is also red and hot.

CRYING

Crying is normal and to be expected as the child expands his lungs and expresses some of the inevitable frustrations of life. There is usually a clear-cut cause:- such as, discomfort from a wet or full nappy, hunger, wind, colic, teething, an infection, or frustration and anger at being held in check.

Only if crying is persistent and recurrent does it become a problem, usually a sign that the mother has not fully understood the needs of the child, he has not taken enough milk from the breast, or the child is developing colicky pains because of something the child is allergic to. The commonest causes are cow's milk, orange juice, or something the breast-feeding mother is eating, e.g. raw onions, which passes into the milk and does not agree with the child.

Of course the child will also cry if he has fallen and hurt himself, is in pain, or where he is being abused. In most cases, the problem can be resolved easily by examining why the crying happens, and what aggravates it (and also relieves it). Your health visitor will also give advice on how to handle this particular problem.

Remedies to consider:

Carbo veg

For the child who is flabby weak and listless, crying from boredom and fatigue. The child is never really well with a weak digestive system, flatulence and acidity.

Chamomilla

Here the child is restless, irritable and attention-seeking, demanding to be held or played with constantly and cries from rage because he feels neglected or abandoned.

Pulsatilla

For tearful behaviour in a passive, shy ,insecure child who is worse for heat and any emotional situation. There is often a mixture of flight and provocative attention-seeking behaviour.

Sulphur

The child is untidy and ill-organised in most things including his feelings. There may be attacks of crying because he is frustrated at being unable to resolve a problem, but much of the time he lacks persistence and confidence, quickly leaving a problem he cannot solve in a short time. Painful colicky indigestion from excess food intake is a common problem.

CUTS, BRUISES, GRAZES

These are an inevitable part of life's learning process, especially for the young child who spends the first year of life trying to become proficient at crawling, climbing and walking. Falls, bruises and little cuts are inevitable and are best dealt with by the mother herself, unless more severe damage has occurred.

It is usually best to expose to the air a small cut or graze without covering it. In this way it will quickly dry and form a natural barrier to infection with the scab. This should not be removed, but allowed to fall off naturally after a week or two.

If the cut is deep, it should be gently washed with warm water, and covered with a plaster, after any dirt, glass or foreign material, has been carefully removed.

If in doubt about any remaining foreign material, take the child to the local casualty department. A tetanus vaccination is usually recommended where the wound has contained soil, or if it is very dirty.

Homoeopathic creams are available to soothe superficial grazed or cut areas of skin. Those containing Arnica, Calendula, or Rhus tox are especially useful. If the damage is more severe, results are usually better with the oral tablets or pills, rather than with a cream. A homoeopathic cream or ointment can be used concurrently with an oral preparation.

Remedies to consider:

Aconitum
For acute painful skin grazes, the child fearful and very restless, sometimes with acute emotional shock from fear. All symptoms are worse for cold air or extremes of heat.

Apis
For swollen, red inflamed areas, which irritate or sting, the child restless, weak and tearful.

Arnica
This remedy promotes healing where there is soreness, damage and bruising with inflammation in the nerve and circulatory systems under the skin.

Calendula
A major remedy to stimulate repair and healing by forming healthy granulation tissue to heal cuts and grazes and all damage to skin tissue.

Rhus tox
For mild, irritating bruised or cut skin areas, usually red and swollen, worse for cold and damp, better for rubbing and heat.

DEAFNESS

This may be congenital or associated with nerve damage from infection, trauma, or sometimes due to simple blockage of the external ear by wax or a foreign body. Every young child should be routinely given a hearing check by the health visitor between seven to nine months, to ensure that normal hearing is present.

If deafness is suspected, in one or both ears, it should be discussed with the health visitor or your doctor. Depending upon the age of the child, an audiogram or test of hearing at different frequencies will probably be recommended.

When deafness is due to infection this can usually be treated with a full recovery. If a foreign body is suspected, the child should be taken to the casualty department for examination and removal. Often an offensive smell comes from the ear which is blocked, alerting the parent to the cause of the deafness and usually discomfort.

Whenever there is a hearing problem, this needs a full and proper diagnosis of the causes. The deaf child often requires a series of specialised hearing tests, also help in a special hearing clinic. If the degree of deafness is severe, he may require help with a hearing aid. As always in homoeopathy, the treatment is determined by the cause and the individual.

Remedies to consider:

Aconitum   For transient deafness associated with acute infection of the throat and ear, often due to an acute cold.

Phosphorus For the thin, active, nervous child with hearing problems. Sounds re-echo and he has problems when there is background noise.

Pulsatilla For variable deafness associated with sinus congestion.

DELAYED DEVELOPMENTAL MILESTONES

This can occur because of an unhealthy pregnancy and a low birth weight, associated with smoking by the mother.

A low birth weight may mean that all the developmental processes are delayed. Other factors are environmental:- lead pollution, possibly high levels of dust, sulphur dioxide or carbon monoxide in the air. The child is unhealthy and slow in all his growth steps.

The cause may be due to a condition of hormonal balance or metabolism, as occurs when there is a thyroid goitre (swelling) or a malfunctioning of the adrenal gland. These may be associated with a genetic abnormality.

Where the quality of fresh food and balanced nutrition is unsatisfactory, this also acts as a brake to growth.

Plenty of holding, home play with lively chatter is essential for the child to expand and develop. This should be from the immediate family and relatives, also friends outside the family to give the child a varied environmental experience and stimulus to growth. He should also have lots of contact with other children..

There is usually a very positive response to homoeopathy.

Remedies to consider:

Baryta carb   For the small underdeveloped child, slow in all his milestones, with problems of chronic catarrh, sensitive to cold air. The child may be mentally as well as physically retarded.

Calcarea   For the pale, weak, slow child, lacking in confidence and with obsessional tendencies. Sinus problems and colds are common. There may be head sweats at night, the pillow sometimes drenched with perspiration.

Silicea   The child is thin, pale, underweight, with unpleasant foot sweating and a tendency for all cuts to fester and heal slowly.

DIARRHOEA

An irritable bowel upset with loose and watery stools is commonly the result of indigestion, the food not agreeing with the child for some reason, often because it was taken too fast or the child is allergic to it. A common example is intolerance of cow's milk leading to vomiting, gastric flatulence and diarrhoea. With an older child it may be caused by infected food, lack of hygiene in preparation, too much taken too quickly, or the food is excessively rich or acidic for the intestine.

If the child has a temperature, give fluids only until the temperature is normal. If normal, give a light diet, little and often, as long as it is easy to digest, letting the child state what he wants to eat. Meals should not be spicy, rich, or potentially irritating. If you suspect an infection, take stricter hygiene precautions with clothes and washing hands after cleaning up the child, as an infection can quickly spread, and involve the whole family. Make sure that the young baby does not get dehydrated. The symptoms to look for are a sunken soft spot on the head, reduced urinary output, the nappies still dry after six hours, the skin loose and lacking elasticity and moisture. If a young child has a diarrhoea problem, give plenty of clear fluids - breast, bottle or cup, in small amounts, but always frequently and avoid giving him cow's milk or formula milk for a 24 hour period. But if the baby is under four months of age, consult your doctor or health visitor first, before restricting the milk intake. If vomiting occurs as well as diarrhoea, dehydration may occur very rapidly and parents should always observe the child closely. If diarrhoea persists for more than 24 hours, especially with a young baby, get a medical opinion.

Remedies to consider :

Arsenicum

Watery diarrhoea, dark in colour and foul-smelling. There may be blood in the stool. The child is usually chilly and shuns company. Weakness and exhaustion are a characteristic sign for this remedy with intense feelings of coldness and desire for heat such as a hot water bottle.

Phosphoric acid

Useful where there is an acute painless or recurrent diarrhoea, the stool yellow, sometimes covered with slime.

Podophyllum

There is a severe watery offensive-smelling diarrhoea accompanied by a secretion of mucus on the stool, colicky abdominal pain, nausea and vomiting.

Sulphur

The child feels too hot. The diarrhoea is gassy and offensive and often chronic. Hunger for fatty or sweet foods persists despite the symptoms which are typically worse on waking.

DISLOCATION

Usually a congenital abnormality, the joint capsule too lax and especially involving the hip. Trauma from the birth, especially with a difficult or sometimes inexperienced forceps delivery, can lead to dislocation, usually of the shoulder.

In all cases the dislocation must be corrected, the bone replaced back correctly in position within the joint capsule by an experienced orthopaedic paediatric surgeon or physician.

After re-positioning, a plaster cast is usually applied. At this stage, homoeopathy can be effectively used to reduce swelling, pain and discomfort. Dislocation of the clavicle or collar bone may also occur, usually from trauma or a fall.

Dislocation of the hip of a young baby is routinely checked for as soon as the baby is born and is often screened for by the general practitioner during the first year of life.

Remedies to consider :

Arnica

There is shock and bruised pain. The remedy is indicated to reduce swelling and inflammation after surgical re-positioning and correction of the dislocation.

Bellis Perennis

A major remedy for ligament and nerve injury or bruising. The area feels chilled,bruised, worse for cold air or water on the affected joint area.

Calcarea

Both child and joints are weak and flabby. Because the supportive joint ligaments are weak, there is a tendency for repeated dislocation to occur.

DRUG DEPENDENCY - MOTHER OR BABY

Drug dependency is still a major social problem in our time, worse in the U.S. but also present as a significant risk factor in Europe and the U.K. By far the greatest risk for the mother and child are the drugs of abuse and dependency, especially Heroin, Cocaine, or Methadrine and the young child is particularly vulnerable.

Any drug taken in pregnancy, may put the foetus at risk but also undermine the future health of the child. Prescribed tranquillisers, or sedatives for sleeping problems are undesirable in pregnancy and may later undermine the mother-child bonding relationship.

Equally dangerous are the social dependent drugs and habits. Alcohol is a risk to the foetus and smoking by the mother both during and after pregnancy.

Coffee and tea-drinking are social props which damage health when taken to excess. Both are undesirable during pregnancy, when breast-feeding and affect the young child because they undermine health. The child may also dragged down by the jaded health of the mother.

Any form of drug dependency is undesirable and psychologically weakening, whatever form it takes. Every mother should aim to avoid all forms of addiction. She should always ensure that psychologically she sets the right example for her child, but also keeping his diet balanced and healthy, not allowing him tea, coffee or alcohol. In this way she can help to ensure that his future health is already started in childhood and kept to an optimum.

Remedies to consider:

Avena sat Where drugs are taken as an escape from extremes of exhaustion, insomnia and lack of concentration. The drug problem may have begun with an initial alcohol dependence.

Nux vomica For dependency problems associated with extremes of intense mood-changes with irritability and usually spasms of pain from either constipation or indigestion.

Pulsatilla For a dependent weak and passive personality, seeking approval, too easily led and influenced by others. All moods and emotions are changeable and unpredictable.

Silicea There is lack of self-will and confidence causing a drifting into drug abuse. The child is vulnerable because he is unsure of himself, lacking drive, purpose and self-trust.

DUMMIES

These are not recommended because they can deform the jaw and retard bite development or distort tooth positioning. They increase the likelihood of infection occurring, particularly of the mouth, lips and facial skin area. Dummies are unhygienic, they are largely unnecessary, and create an undesirable habit. It may interfere with the natural development of language which starts as soon as the child is born, when the free spontaneous expression of each sound or noise the child makes is very important.

The regular use of a dummy may reinforce unhealthy psychological habits (passive oral dependency) in later life, leading to, eating, smoking, tobacco or gum chewing and eventually obesity, when under pressure, or there is a problem or frustration, rather than resolving it.

The device may encourage passivity in the adult. Instead of patiently putting up with a situation, he should be more complaining about it, or much more active and positive, expressing himself in a more assertive individual way.

Some modern dummies are marketed as less damaging to the mouth and teeth, than the earlier models, but in the main they are undesirable and should be discouraged from the start.

HOMOEOPATHY AND INDIVIDUALITY *

Homoeopathy is more than just an effective treatment for the individual, it is an overall way of looking at the patient. Every aspect of the person is taken into account when assessing and considering the most appropriate remedy for a problem, and one likely to help. However physical the complaint - perhaps a problem of eczema, hiatus hernia, blood-pressure, varicose veins, or haemorrhoids, the patient's psyche and psychological make-up is always considered in detail, as part of understanding the totality of the illness and totality of the person.

Homoeopathy's major concern is stimulation of the individual's overall response, and a more balanced functioning of the internal organs to build-up vitality and reserves. This overall functioning of the patient is taken into account each time a remedy is prescribed, with attention to both physical and psychological areas of concern or pre-occupation for the individual.

But homoeopathy is more than just a simple treatment of illness, it is also an effective diagnostic approach to the individual as a unique entity in his own right, based on how the person is feeling at the time, in the consulting room *now*, and not in a remote past situation. Remedies are about curing present-day problems, and are diagnosed by the symptoms and awareness of the patient as he is evolving and changing.

Every patient is more than just a collection of symptoms and clinical signs. He is also a human being with feelings, sensitivity and vulnerability.
* From Understanding Homoeopathy

EAR INFECTION

One of the most common and painful of all the childhood infections. It is frequently very acute and accompanied by a high temperature. The cause is often unknown, but it usually follows an acute throat cold, or tonsillitis, sometimes is a local infection from swimming in the sea, or a pool which has not been disinfected. It may be an external otitis (the outer part of the ear only is infected), or involving the middle ear, inside the drum (otitis media).

External otitis is usually less painful and often a more chronic problem with redness and an oozing from the infected area. A local rash, sometimes flaking and irritating is present in the area affected. The cause may be bacterial or viral, but it is often fungal in origin.

Otitis media or middle ear infection may be bacterial or viral. It is extremely painful and the body temperature is usually high, the child restless with disagreeable acute pain. If pressure within the middle ear is raised, the drum may burst, with a discharge of foul-smelling matter, sometimes of pus, which relieves the pain. The drum normally heals completely and spontaneously with no after-effects.

Remedies to consider:

Aconitum

For acute conditions, within the first 48 hours of infection, the ear hot and painful, the child restless and fearful.

Antimonium crud

For more acute infections, the ear and surrounding area, red with a thick yellow ear discharge, the local lymph glands tender to touch.

Belladonna

For acutely painful ear infections, the ear and often surrounding area of the face, red and hot with a high fever, the child restless and anxious.

Hepar sulph

For acute conditions, the pain is sharp and stabbing, aggravated from lying on the side affected. This is a very useful remedy to consider in a low 6c potency. Irritability is marked.

Pulsatilla

The infection is less acute and variable, with a yellowish or green catarrhal discharge. All symptoms are worse for heat but better for fresh air. The child is usually very tearful.

Pyrogen

For acute ear conditions with restlessness and a high fever.

ECZEMA

This is a common and usually transient problem for a young baby or child. It is often of allergic origin, typically due to a cleansing product or soap that the child reacts to. Similarly he could react to a particular food or household pet. Often the cause is unknown, but at least one of the parents have usually had eczema as a child or adult. The condition varies in extent and severity, but typically involves the flexure crease areas of the body, especially the wrist and knee, also the face, scalp and limbs. The eczema rash is variable, and may be moist or dry, crack or flake. Eczema is always distressing to the child and whenever possible it should be treated early, not left to become a chronic problem. Parents should at all times keep the child's delicate skin soft and hydrated, using a simple unperfumed moisturising lotion or cream, such as Calendula or aqueous cream, to prevent the skin drying or cracking, which may lead to infection. Bubble bath or any toilet product, such as soap, which dries the skin should be avoided. Clothing which irritates or rubs, especially nylon or a harsh wool, should be replaced with cotton. If the eczema is food-related, parents should balance the effects on the child's skin, with the effects of a restricted diet on the child's development. At times the mother may feel guilty or depressed,or a failure because of the child's eczema, interfering with the early bonding process, or isolating him from other children and social contacts. If left untreated; the child may scratch at night, interfering with sleep, tired and irritable during the day, failing to stay alert at playgroup or in class, causing a reduction in educational attainments and undermining social skills and confidence.

Remedies to consider:

Graphites
The eczema tends to crack and ooze a clear, sticky pale yellow discharge, especially behind the ears. Most symptoms are better if covered with a dry dressing but aggravated by any form of heat.

House dust
The dry, red and intensely itching eczema is associated with an aggravation after contact with house-dust, following dusting or cleaning, usually due to allergy to the house-dust mite.

Petroleum
For a dry, rough, intensely irritating eczema which tends to crack or bleed. It is often aggravated by cold weather and tends to chap easily in winter.

Rhus tox
The skin is raised, red and irritated, better for a warm application and aggravated by any form of chill or cold.

Sulphur
For chronic eczema problems with irritable burning recurrent areas of infection which quickly suppurate. The skin looks grubby and dirty-looking. There is intolerance of water, dislike of washing and any form of heat.

EYE PROBLEMS

These often occur in a young child or baby. They are quite common after birth due to mild infection or a blocked tear-duct which does not allow proper drainage of the eye. They are often helped by wiping the eye clean with a weak saline solution - one grain of salt in boiled water in an eye bath and allowed to cool.

CONJUNCTIVITIS

Inflammation or irritation of the delicate conjunctival layer of the eye, causing redness, watering and irritation. It may be due to a draught of cold air, local infection, repetitive rubbing, dust, or a small insect in the corner of the eye. Other causes are general allergic reactions, as hay-fever, also during measles. Children should be discouraged from rubbing their eye, as this may lead to infection.

STICKY EYE

An infection in the corner of one eye, is often self-inflicted by rubbing the eye, but also linked to low resistance in the child. There may have been frequent infections at this time:- including colds, chest infections, sinus catarrh, problems of environmental dust, noise, or air pollution, often with inadequate natural sunlight. All of these factors, when combined with an inadequate diet, may cause the condition.

BLACK EYE

The typical discolouration is due to breakage of small vessels under the skin which leak blood into the surrounding tissues. There is no eye damage and pain or tenderness responds well to homoeopathy. An ice pack also helps to reduce the swelling.

Remedies to consider:

Antimonium crud   There is a painful irritating thick discharge of pus from the infected eye, the child irritable and restless.

Arnica   The eye is sore and feels tender, painful and bruised.

Belladonna   For acute conjunctivitis, the eye red, swollen and painful.

China   For mild sticky eye problems, the child lifeless, the eye sore from draughts of cold air.

Euphrasia   For problems of conjunctivitis, with redness, irritation and constant watering.

Gelsemium   For problems of focusing, the eyes tired and heavy.

Hamamelis   For bruised soreness, with considerable venous congestion and discolouration.

Ledum   For bruising, the surrounding area chilled, worse for heat, better for a cold compress.

Ruta   For eye-strain or eye tiredness from long periods of close work, the eyes, red and irritated.

FAILURE TO THRIVE

Whenever a baby or child fails to develop to its full potential, in size and body weight for its age, it is a problem that must be taken seriously and a full diagnosis made of the underlying causes. Because every baby is vulnerable if it is underweight and small, it is essential to start treatment as soon as the problem is fully understood, to help the child build up strength and resistance quickly.

The most common reason for failure to thrive is that the diet is insufficient, particularly where a baby is breast fed, the milk supply usually inadequate. In some parts of the world, famine is endemic and there is insufficient food available for the mother and child. Other dietary causes are where a child is kept for too long on the bottle and given cow's milk or a milk formula without supplements, then the child becomes anaemic and undernourished. Intolerance of a certain type of food in the diet is a frequent cause of the baby not gaining weight, especially intolerance of cow's milk or gluten. Other causes are either physical or psychological. The physical causes are congenital abnormality involving a major organ, particularly the heart, but also the kidneys or neurological system may be concerned. Infection such as syphilis or tuberculosis can be the underlying problem, also drug addiction of the newborn, AIDS, or any acute infection such as cholera or dysentery.

Psychological causes are sometimes relevant, usually where there is conflict within the family and a separation or divorce has occurred. If a parent has died, this may leave the both partner and the child depressed.

Remedies to consider :

Baryta carb   For the child who is small, weak and slow, mentally and physically retarded at all his expected milestones. Lack of energy and drive is marked. He tends to suffer from chronic sinus or nasal catarrhal problems.

Calcarea   For the chilly overweight sluggish child, often ritualistic or obsessional and lacking in drive and energy. There is a marked tendency to sweat, especially about the head at night.

Silicea   For thin small underweight and undersized children, who lack drive and confidence. They tend to sweat offensively, particularly on the feet. Because they are low on vitality and resistance, every cut or graze becomes infected.

Tuberculinum   For thin hyperactive children who are slow to grow and thrive. They often have a chronic dry cough. There may be a history of tuberculosis in a distant member of the family, or there may have been a past contact or infection by one of the parents or grandparents.

FEEDING PROBLEMS

Where there are feeding difficulties with a young baby or child, these are often best discussed with the health visitor. She will observe the mother feeding the child or preparing his meals and give practical advice on techniques and how best to approach the problem. Often the cause is either inexperience by the mother, or anxiety and panic when the child either cries or does not take the food given.

Often the food has not been properly prepared or presented so that it is appetizing and acceptable to the child. In many cases the child is being given cow's milk where there is an intolerance to this type of food. This is now well understood and healthy well-formulated soya milk substitutes are available which are well tolerated by the child. A very young baby should not however be put on a soya-based formula milk without first discussing this with your doctor or health visitor. Because of high aluminium levels, which may be detrimental to the child's development, a soya-based formula milk should if possible be avoided for the first six weeks.

In other instances, either insufficient food is given for the needs of the child and he cries because he is hungry, or too much is given too quickly without winding the baby, so that he vomits or regurgitates. When this happens the baby cries because he is full of wind, in discomfort, and hungry at the same time. If this happens, it is essential to take more time giving the feed, and to wind the baby frequently. If the mother is tense and anxious, this makes for a tense and anxious child.

Remedies to consider:

Aethusa

Due to milk intolerance, there are problems of colicky pains with nausea, mucus production and vomiting after feeding.

Lycopodium

The child is usually anxious and insecure, all problems worse in the late afternoon and early evening, with flatulence and wind, aggravated by a high intake of carbohydrates. Constipation is a major problem and cause of discomfort.

Pulsatilla

For fair, shy and tearful children, with changeable feeding problems, especially when intolerant of carbohydrates. The child usually feels worse from heat but better for cool fresh air.

FIRST AID FOR BURNS AND SHOCK

It is common for most children to experience some form of minor burn or scald during their developmental life and unless severe, most mothers can easily treat these safely and simply at home with the appropriate homoeopathic remedies. If the burn or scald is at all severe, or the child is shocked, (pale, weak, sweating, with a slow, thin pulse), the child should be wrapped, kept warm, but not over-heated, and taken to the nearest casualty or burns unit, preferably where there is a paediatric wing for the specialised treatment of young children. Unless the burn is large, try to keep the area dry and exposed to the air. Apply a sterile dressing if the area is large, weeping profusely, or infected. Following a scald, wet clothing should be removed as soon as possible, the scalded area immersed in cool water, poured slowly over the area, until the intense pain passes. Remove any clothing of a tight constrictive nature. After a burn, if the clothing is dry but charred, it can be left in place, as it is sterilized by the heat of the burn. If a burn has been caused by contact with chemicals, such as household caustic cleansers, remove all clothing and wash the affected skin area with plenty of water.

The best treatment is prevention, training children from an early age to be aware of dangers in the home, avoiding playing or standing on chairs near to a stove where there are overhanging saucepan handles. Children should be warned of the dangers of sitting too close to an oven, hot iron, or fire. All household chemical cleansers, oven, drain, or toilet, caustic foam substances, should be stored in a locked cupboard. Fit fire-guards on all fires and sources of direct heat.

Remedies to consider:

Aconitum   For acute first-aid conditions with shock, fear and restlessness, the area swollen and painful.

Arnica   For shock, and bruised, painful, black and blue areas, as after a fall or sprain.

Calendula   A valuable general remedy which promotes the healing of damaged skin and underlying tissue, by promoting increased circulation in the area and repair by supporting the formation of granulation tissue.

Cantharis   Where there are bruised, grazed areas of the body which sting and burn.

Hypericum   A valuable remedy for deeper nerve damage, especially crush injuries, as with a finger caught in the door. Throbbing pain with swelling and redness is common.

Urtica urens   A remedy for burns and scalds, with stinging pain, redness, swelling of the area and intense irritation.

GRUMBLING APPENDIX

This is usually a mild recurrent condition which responds well to homoeopathy. There is lower abdominal pain, usually right-sided without a temperature, nausea or vomiting.

Typical symptoms are recurring colicky pains, sometimes a little diarrhoea and worse after meals or exercise. Young children may experience griping tummy pains, or stitch-like discomfort with nausea, mainly situated in the lower abdomen. At times the child may feel quite unwell with the discomfort, typically looking pale and feeling sick.

Provided that the child remains well and is not toxic (obviously ill and exhausted, or confused, with a raised temperature), or in a collapsed state (pale, fainting, or weak and often sweating), the abdomen soft to the touch and not hard or rigid, then homoeopathy can be safely given.

Should the abdomen become hard; the temperature elevated, the child in severe pain, or obviously ill and weak, he should be taken to the local casualty department to exclude an acute appendicitis which may require surgical treatment.

Remedies to consider:

Lycopodium For painful abdominal conditions, usually recurrent, often worse in the afternoon and early evening. The discomfort is usually right-sided, associated with flatulence and a sense of fullness. Most symptoms are worse after eating, often after a small meal and leading to pain and discomfort. The pain is usually better for warmth, such as a hot water bottle to the abdominal area.

Magnesia phos A useful remedy for griping colicky pains, doubling the child up, better for rubbing and warmth, but not relieved by bringing up wind. The child feels tired and exhausted.

Nux vomica For spasms of colicky or dull bruised lower abdominal pain, also distention with tenderness. There is often nausea or vomiting, the child constipated and usually irritable. Most symptoms are worse from food and in the mornings.

INFECTION

All children will inevitably be infected by some organism during their school and pre-school years. The most frequent is the common cold, but a sore throat, acute ear problem, skin, or sinus infections are frequent.

Most infections are minor in the healthy child and the best prevention is to help the child to be well both physically and psychologically. In this way when an infection does occur, it is usually a relatively minor affair and does not require antibiotic treatment.

More rarely, a serious acute illness occurs and involves the chest:- with bronchitis or pneumonia, the brain membranes with meningitis or encephalitis, the kidney with pyelitis.

In many of these, the infection is of a very virulent type and often other cases occur in the same school or neighbourhood. The acute bacterial or viral illnesses of childhood, such as, measles, mumps, or whooping cough, are other examples of more generalised forms of infection.

Where a child is weak, or convalescent, or another condition is affecting the immune system (for example:- HIV infection), or the child is taking a course of steroids, any infection may be much more serious, and extra care is required.

Remedies to consider:

Antimonium crud   For severe localised infective conditions with a thick yellow or white discharge, often painless and worse for heat or cold applications. The child is usually very irritable.

Arsenicum   For acute infective conditions, especially of the chest or abdomen. There is often a severe cough with shortness of breath or wheezing, usually worse after midnight.

Hepar Sulph   For less acute and more localised infective conditions, especially of the throat, with sharp splinter or stitch-like pains. They are very sensitive to draughts of cold air and better for warmth.

Nux vomica   For spasms of pain, with severe constipation and irritability. Nausea or vomiting is common.

Pulsatilla   For milder variable infective problems, associated with mood changes, aggravated by excitement or emotion.

Pyrogenium   There is a high temperature, with burning pains, and an offensive discharge.

INSOMNIA

Some sleeping problems are to be expected with a young and hungry baby. Most babies require at least one feed during the night for a few months until they settle into a daytime feeding pattern and are more able to sleep through the night. But again each child is different with differing needs from the start and just as some babies sleep the night through without any need for a feed, others are equally difficult and restless; often with no obvious cause that can be found except individuality and differing hunger patterns. If the problem is due to wind, then this can be easily remedied. It is also important to be sure that the young baby is not too hot and over-wrapped, especially during the summer or in a centrally heated bedroom. It is best to keep the baby on the cool side, rather than over-heated. For a young baby, light cotton bed linen and clothes are preferable. Colic and wind are the most common reasons for the baby not sleeping after hunger (also see the Overactivity section on page 124).

Sometimes a child is not sleeping because it is overactive and has been restless and excitable during the day. The problem is often more stressful for the parents than the child, and they often become very tired, irritable and feel ambivalent towards the baby or child, however much they love him. Try to have a quiet period with the baby or young child before settling him to sleep. Make sure that you are calm and unruffled, enjoying the child and also relaxed. The baby will soon pick this up and relax with you, which in itself encourages sleep. Ensure that you give the baby lots of calm attention before he sleeps, and that he is not excited by another child, or in contact with stress or noise just before he is due to sleep (also see page 144).

Remedies to consider:

Arsenicum   The child wakes up cold and feeling anxious, between midnight and 1.00am. He is often agitated, but does not like a lot of fuss or attention. Chesty colds are a frequent problem.

Coffea   For inability to get off to sleep because the mind is overactive. The child is excitable, often complaining of palpitations, heartburn, or stomach cramps. He may sweat profusely.

Lycopodium   For inability to get off to sleep, the child too excitable, but also anxious, usually worried about something that may or is about to happen in the future. He also lacks confidence.

Passiflora   Useful for sleep problems where the child is over-tired or exhausted so that he cannot easily relax. Useful where there has been stress in the family provoking anxiety, or the child has been under much pressure.

Pulsatilla   For variable changeable sleep patterns. The child wakes hungry, feeling too hot, yet desiring a warm drink or something to eat.

JEALOUSY PROBLEMS

Some jealousy is normal for every child, especially sibling rivalry and sibling jealousy. Every child wants to feel special, to be the most loved and wanted one, but at the same time fears that it is another sibling, sometimes a parent or live-in partner, who is most important to the mother.

Jealousy is mainly unnecessary and destructive. It can be avoided if the mother ensures that her child is made to feel valued and special, but not more than another child in the family. In this way all the family are made to feel valued for their own uniqueness and individuality.

The child should be made to feel that he is no less important because he is older or younger, boy or girl, less intelligent than another sibling, less attractive, or less inclined towards sport, games or play.

Whenever insecurity is spotted by the parents accompanied by feelings of jealousy, it should be given immediate thought, taken up and discussed with the individual child as soon as possible.

Remedies to consider:

Lachesis

For problems of mistrust, lack of confidence and jealousy. All the symptoms are worse on waking and aggravated by sleep.

Lycopodium

For the child who appears more secure, older and mature than he is in reality, and it is this pseudo-maturity which creates many of the emotional problems which beset him.

Pulsatilla

For the insecure, frightened, easily panicky child who is always running away from life and comparing himself unfavourably with others - hence the jealousy and the fears of anything new in his life. Sudden shifts of emotion with floods of tears changing to peals of laughter are characteristic.

Sulphur

The child is often as untidy in his mind as with his clothes and personal belongings. Everything tends to be poorly organised and badly co-ordinated, which leads him to put too much emphasis on others, idealising them, at the same time also idealising his own scattered thoughts and fantasies.

MEASLES

The most common infectious disease of children. Following contact there is an incubation period of 8 to 14 days before symptoms develop. It is now a relatively mild illness. The complications which occur are a middle ear infection (otitis media), pneumonia, rarely encephalitis (inflammation of the brain).

Initially the condition starts with symptoms of a cold, with a sore throat, mild conjunctivitis (red eye) and a dry irritating cough. At this stage tiny white spots like grains of salt can be observed on the child's throat and inside the mouth, on the inner cheek area. The rash occurs on the 4th day, initially behind the ears, then spreading, with a red blotchy irritating rash over the whole body. The child only feels mildly ill, the throat sore.

It is helpful to keep the temperature down by sponging the child and giving the appropriate homoeopathic remedy. The child should be kept quiet, with plenty of fluids and a light diet. Bathe the eyes with a dilute saline solution.

Children are routinely vaccinated against Measles, (together with Mumps and German Measles), in their second year of life, and this helps to give some protection against a severe form of the disease developing. In most cases, a Measles infection is not serious, and the child feels better within a few days.

Remedies to consider:

Baryta Carb   There is a sore throat with tender lymphatic neck glands, especially when the child is weak, convalescent, or growth is retarded in any way.

Morbillinum   The specific homoeopathic vaccine-equivalent nosode.

Pulsatilla   All symptoms are variable, the child often miserable, tearful, complaining of being too hot. He is easily chilled, but better for fresh air, and open windows.

Rhus tox   The main problem is the rash, with itchy swollen spots containing a clear fluid. The child is sensitive to touch, and feels better for the local warmth.

Sulphur   The rash is oozing or discharging. The throat is infected, all symptoms worse for heat or contact with water.

MOUTH ULCERS

These are common and often viral in origin associated with a child who is under par, with resistance and vitality at a low level, usually because the child is unwell from some other cause or is convalescent or tired.

In some cases, the parents also have mouth ulcers and when this happens, direct mouth to mouth contact should be avoided until the condition clears. A dilute saline mouthwash, or the direct local application to the mouth ulcer of dilute (1 part in 100) Potassium permanganate can also be helpful.

Every attempt should be made to improve the general health and resistance of the child by giving a healthier balanced diet with plenty of fresh vegetables and fruit. Fresh air and taking the child for regular exercise in a healthy area away from dust and pollution is to be encouraged.

Remedies to consider:

Natrum mur   For chronic mouth ulcer problems, the child lacking vitality and with a lowered resistance, often craving salt. There are frequently underlying emotional problems which are a drain on health.

Nitric acid   For painful mouth ulcer problems, with sharp burning or splinter-like pains in the area affected. The child is usually irritable and most symptoms are worse in the evening and from heat.

Sulphur   For more chronic problems, the whole skin area irritated or infected. The child is usually overweight, all symptoms aggravated by heat.

MUMPS

The common, highly infective, acute viral illness of childhood has an incubation period of 14 to 21 days. It usually begins with infection of one of the salivary glands around the jaw, with pain and swelling of one side of the face. The main symptom is a dry mouth with often severe discomfort on opening the mouth or swallowing. There is no typical rash present as in measles. The child is initially unwell, with a slightly raised temperature. The condition usually spontaneously subsides over a period of 3 to 4 weeks.

Vaccination is carried out routinely in the second year, (together with Measles, Mumps, and German Measles), to help reduce the incidence and severity of these infections, but consider a homoeopathic alternative approach if you are unhappy about this, or where orthodox vaccination is contra-indicated (see page 178).

Complications sometimes occur, with meningitis, the child developing a high temperature, irritability and neck stiffness on about the tenth day after the acute illness has subsided.

Rarely the mumps virus is passed to an adult member of the family. In the male it may involve the testicle and cause swelling and pain (orchitis), occasionally resulting in sterility. If an adult woman is affected it may involve the breast glandular tissue causing a painful mumps mastitis.

Reassurance is important during the acute stages of the illness, and if the throat is very painful, give the child plenty of cool fluids, if necessary through a straw.

Remedies to consider:

Baryta carb The throat is acutely infected, red and tight. Swallowing is painful, the parotid lymphatic gland swollen and painful, the child nervous, weak and anxious with low assertiveness and lacking confidence.

Parotidinum The specific mumps nosode or homoeopathic vaccine-equivalent.

Pulsatilla For variable symptoms, the swelling and throat, worse for warmth and taking fluid. There is loss of thirst, although the child complains of being too hot and then suddenly chilled. Tearful and very changeable moods are characteristic.

NAPPY RASH

Every child develops a nappy rash at some time during its development and parents should not feel guilty or that they have failed to care for the child properly when it occurs. The most common cause is a bacterial reaction from a 'dirty' nappy, acting on urine which is frequently passed by the young baby.

The sealing-in of infected acid urine within the nappy, causes ammonia to be released, breaking down the natural skin barrier and tending to burn and irritate the buttock skin area. The skin becomes red and may then become infected by bacteria present.

Prevention is usually the best approach. Exposing the nappy area to fresh air for half an hour twice daily is especially useful, also using a thin barrier cream over the entire nappy area can be of help.

Change a 'dirty' nappy as soon as possible, and if nappy rash does occur, despite the preventative steps mentioned, expose the skin to fresh air for longer periods, and use a cream, such as Calendula to help heal the skin. Consider discarding all nappies until the rash has resolved. In this way, it usually clears within a few days.

Calendula, or a simple moisturising cream, helps to relieve irritation and makes the rash more comfortable for the baby. The use of even small amounts of a proprietary drug, steroid-based cream or ointment, on the area, may lead to some degree of drug absorption into the general system of the child, with the risk of side-effects, especially on a young baby.

Remedies to consider:

Antimonium crud There is a painful, tender infected rash, the skin dry and irritated, aggravated by heat and from washing, but better if left exposed to cool air.

Belladonna The rash is dry and red. The area feels hot, is irritable and itching. All symptoms are aggravated by heat or water.

Calendula Useful as a local cream or ointment application. It should only be used sparingly when it encourages healing.

Cantharis Of value where the skin area is particularly irritated with burning, scalding, irritation, aggravated by any touching or from cold water.

Mercurius The skin is red, sore, irritable, with multiple small painful infected spots.

Rhus tox The area is raised, red and irritated, always better for local warmth and when the child is running around.

Sulphur For long-term chronic nappy rash problems, the area dirty-looking, with a low-grade infection.

NIGHT TERRORS

These are often an extension of nightmares and the same underlying psychological causes usually apply. The child is frightened of the dark, going to sleep, being alone, any noise, falling asleep and having a dream. He is often restless and in an agitated state needing comfort, holding and reassurance. Always try to see the underlying psychological problem which is causing anxiety or panic and discuss this with the child as you understand and perceive it. But put it in simple language at the child's level, not in sophisticated adult talk, which will only be more of a threat to the child.

Try not to panic or be anxious yourself. See what is happening as a natural reaction to the child's insecurity and fear of something unknown which threatens him. If the mother stays calm and does not become anxious or panic, because of the child's emotional reactions, this helps the child's confidence and often the severity of the problem.

In most cases the causes of the night terrors are perfectly understandable and there is an acute crisis within the family, or a communications problem that has been left and is causing tension. The child senses the emotional tensions and often the unexpressed aggression or agitation that is present.

Be patient, give the child more individual time and be prepared to listen and understand, to clarify what is happening and why he is fearful. If still in doubt and you are not able to resolve the problem within the family, discuss it with your health visitor or doctor.

Remedies to consider:

Aconitum   For acute night-time anxiety problems, with fears about the future, of death or dying, the child crying, tense and restless. Most of the fears are aggravated by heat and better for fresh air and reassurance.

Argentum nit   For the anxious child with phobic-anxiety problems, lacking in confidence. All the fears are aggravated by heat of any form.

Gelsemium   For milder hysterical types of night-time anxiety, the child wakes wanting reassurance and to climb into the parents bed. The child is very sensitive to any emotion or excitement which aggravates the problem, mainly because of underlying insecurity and lack of confidence.

Natrum mur   For long-standing confidence problems, the child thin, pessimistic and tearful. He is usually a loner, often frightened of playing with other children, and prefers his own company, to play quietly on his own, feeling more secure and especially more in control, when others are not around.

NIGHTMARES

These occur at some time in the life of every child and are a break-through of excitement, anxiety and fear into sleep, often about a new anticipated situation and provoked by the underlying emotion. They are common before starting school for the first time, a change of school, before a holiday and where there is a divorce, separation, or change in the family dynamics of any kind which makes the child feel insecure.

Usually the child needs reassurance, a hug and a cuddle, explaining in simple terms, why the nightmare occurred and perhaps what stimulated it. Only if nightmares are repetitive, the child fearful of going to bed, having the light off, tearful, becoming depressed, or losing confidence, is there cause for concern, when treatment may be indicated. If this happens, the mother should look at any recent emotional upheavals within the family, to see if these were a stimulus to anxiety, also noting if his learning curve has dipped recently.

The mother should also note if the child is fearful about going out, or playing with other children. If a nightmare is part of an overall lack of confidence, she should spend more time helping the child to talk about what is worrying him, but always in a simple unpressurised natural way. If there has been a loss or illness in the family, it is best discussed openly. In this way it does not become locked within the child's psyche and associated with guilt. If the child says he feels unhappy, about a loss, it helps if the mother shares some of her own feelings with the child. In this way she encourages the child to worry less, and not to lock feelings away.

Remedies to consider:

Aconitum   For problems of acute distress or very fearful nightmares, the child terror-struck and convinced of the inevitability of the dream and that some harm will come to him. He is usually tearful and needs considerable reassurance before eventually relaxing.

Belladonna   For acute nightmares, the child is hot, restless and red in the face. Anxiety is aggravated by any form of heat and better for fresh air and reassurance.

Natrum mur   Indicated for recurrent anxiety dreams, associated with an underlying confidence or personality problem.

Nux vomica   For recurrent nightmares when the child wakes and is extremely irritable and aggressive and may be difficult to handle for a time before he calms down. Stomach cramps, sometimes with nausea, are frequently a cause of discomfort. Constipation is typically an ongoing problem, mainly the result of underlying anxiety, impeding the normal bowel peristalsis movements.

NITS

Nits or head lice are a common hygiene problem and may involve any child. The commonest age is under eleven, at a time when the child is in close head contact with their peers, playing, either at school or wherever young children group together. Psychologically the problem is often as distressing for the parents as the child, as they feel that the condition is associated with a 'dirty' household. This is untrue, as often the insect prefers to lay its eggs on a clean head, rather than a dirty one. Lice only live on the head, and try to breed there, laying eggs on the hair follicle close to the scalp, the eggs hatching within 7 to 10 days, depending on the amount of heat transmitted from the scalp. The hatched young insect then feeds by puncturing the scalp and taking small amounts of blood, leaving behind its 'saliva' which is an irritant to the skin causing the child to scratch.

Excessive head scratching is often the first sign which alerts the parent that something is wrong and that the child is infected. Nits do not affect the overall health of the child and apart from being unpleasant are not of great significance. The main symptoms are an itching scalp and sometimes slight bleeding from scratching the area.

Because this is a common, often persistent problem, it is important to have a routine of observing a schoolchild's head once a week to look specifically for head lice. To some extent, it can be controlled by encouraging every child to vigorously brush his hair for a few minutes each evening after returning from school. Orthodox treatment uses a head lice lotion, which may be Pyrethroid-based, killing the eggs as well as the lice parasite.

Remedies to consider:

Rhus tox   The child complains of an itchy irritating scalp which is red and tender. He tends to scratch the affected area. The condition improves with warmth as in summer, but is aggravated by cold.

Sulphur   A very useful remedy for recurrent, itchy scalp problems due to nits. The irritation is aggravated by heat, during the summer and also worse for washing or the application of water.

OBESITY

A fat child is never a healthy child and every attempt should be made from the earliest months to prevent this happening. Some babies are born fat and this is always a matter for concern and careful investigation to exclude problems such as diabetes and hormonal or metabolic disturbance. The majority of children who are overweight are the result of an unbalanced diet, with too much carbohydrate and fat given, the child building up fat within the tissues. Obesity often creates an emotional problem , which can become a vicious circle, as the child may tend to eat even more sweet comfort foods in order to reduce anxiety or stress. In a healthy family, every child should be encouraged to exercise daily, learning from the example set by his parents. If the parents are overweight, the child should not develop the same incorrect dietary habits. This is best prevented by careful attention to his diet from the start, beginning as soon as he is weaned off the bottle or breast.

Always encourage a child to eat fresh fruit and salad each day, to have small wholesome meals of whole grain cereal and fresh quality food, preferably cooked fresh, not frozen or microwaved as a routine.

Where the child is already overweight, encourage him to diet and as parents, set the example. Avoid foods which are high in calories and saturated fat, especially crisps, salty nuts, hamburgers, chocolate, cakes, cheese, cream or butter, substituting low fat milk (not recommended for children under the age of five) or soya milk products. Healthy eating should be part of a thoughtful approach to life from the start.

Remedies to consider:

Calcarea   For the flabby, placid, chilly child, lacking drive and delayed or slow in reaching his milestone targets for growth. Sour catarrhal discharges from the nose and throat are usually present and psychologically obsessional patterns of play and movement tend to be common.

Kali carb   The child is overweight and easily tired or exhausted. He is often chilly and wakes early at 4-5.00am with a sore throat, sharp pains or a chesty cold. Depression, anxiety and lack of confidence are also present.

Sulphur   For the flabby unmotivated child who is always too hot and has an unstoppable voracious appetite for anything in the larder. This is usually because of a very high carbohydrate and fat intake leading to a foul-smelling gassy diarrhoea.Indigestion problems with flatulence is common. Because sugar levels are too high, this causes chronic skin problems or infection.

OVERACTIVITY

The overactive child can be a trial for the mother, as he has an enormous supply of energy and drive, often in contrast to the mother who is tired. He rarely seems to need to relax or sleep like other children.

The cause is often unknown, but a too rapid precipitate passage through the birth canal can cause subtle brain damage, as also anoxia at birth or where the birth process has been too slow and the foetal heart has been under strain. Other reasons are believed to be of a less traumatic kind and related to allergic reactions to additives and colourants in foods. When these have been withdrawn completely from the diet, the overactive child often shows a marked improvement. Where there is emotional tension within the family, a child may also become overactive. An anxious tense mother contributes to the child becoming more anxious and tense and this may cause overactivity.

The problem is initially often best treated and diagnosed within a paediatric unit, as far as possible, to find the exact causes of the overactivity. There is usually no specific conventional treatment and the mother has to pay strict attention to the labelling of all food given to the child, avoiding artificial colourants or preservatives in the diet.

Where the environment is noisy, polluted, dusty, and the quality of the air poor, it is even more important to give children a well-balanced varied healthy diet, with adequate vitamins and minerals obtained from their food, rather than from supplements.

Remedies to consider:

Aconitum
For very acute problems of this type, often with a combination of a high temperature, the child red faced and sweating, with restless anxious behaviour marked by severe inconsolable fear of death, or dying with panic.

Belladonna
For acute overactivity problems associated with an acute infection. The child is hot, red-faced with a dry skin, restless and fearful. The pupils are dilated, the temperature often raised because of throat or ear inflammation.

Hyoscyamus
There is severe uncontrollable restless behaviour with fear and irritable or talkative behaviour. Suspicion with lack of trust may be a major feature.

Natrum mur
A remedy for mild hyperactive problems with anxiety. The child is usually a loner and prefers to play quietly in his room, the behaviour pattern aggravated by the presence of other children.

Stramonium
For more violent forms of hyperactivity with destructive behaviour, constant chatter, mood changes, sadness or depression.

PAIN AND COLIC

These are a common problem for the young baby. Air is sucked in and swallowed as the bottle or breast is sucked. Often the child takes in the milk too quickly or there is too much for it to cope with. The mother must always monitor the amount of food that the child is getting and ensure that the child is not being drowned by too much, too quickly. If this happens it will gulp down both food and air and develop colic.

The baby should be winded regularly, depending upon the particular child, but every five minutes for a young baby. The mother must ensure that the child is not allergic to the milk she is giving and that the breast milk is suiting the child, or does not contain some item of food, such as raw onions, which the mother is eating, then getting into the milk and upsetting the child. For the same reason, it is important that the mother should not be taking any drugs or supplements at this time, unless strictly necessary, as they may upset the baby's digestion.

The mother should be as relaxed as possible and not under pressure when feeding, so that the child feels that it does not have to gulp down and hurry before the bottle or breast is taken away. If the child is allergic to cows milk, as shown by vomiting, and excessive colic or diarrhoea, with failure to gain weight, a soya milk formulation should be tried after discussion with the health visitor.

Rarely there is a medical cause for the colic and where this is suspected, it is important that the child is examined during its feed by the doctor or health visitor.

Remedies to consider:

Aethusa

For colicky pains, restless tearful behaviour, nausea and vomiting associated with marked milk intolerance.

Iris versic

There is severe colic with flatulence.

Magnesium phos

For severe cramping pains which double the child up in an effort to find relief. All cramping symptoms are better for local applied warmth, as from a hot water bottle. The abdominal area is tender, the child resisting any attempt to touch the sensitive area. He is also aggravated by cold drinks or cold air.

Nux vomica

For spasms of colicky pain, in any area of the body. The child is irritable and aggressive, the stools usually constipated. The symptoms are better for warm damp weather but aggravated by cold drinks or weather.

Plumbum met

Violent abdominal colicky pains occur, with numbness or stiffness of the limbs.

Veratrum

Colicky pains, worse at night, the child feeling ice-cold.

PHOBIAS

These are sometimes a problem for the young child and associated with insecurity, often because the child's natural confidence has been undermined by a crisis within the family. In many cases, it is a crisis within the parents relationship, which creates insecurity within the child. Whenever a parent leaves the home during a crisis and separation, it is usual for any child to become more dependent and clinging, frightened of being separated from the remaining parent, especially more nervous at bedtime. Children can easily feel panicky about the dark, about dreams or nightmares, about sleeping alone, or sometimes they feel insecure and frightened on waking. The insecure child can develop fears, which may become severe about things they were previously perfectly confident with or even attracted to. One little girl of 6 developed a fear of spiders, although in the past she had kept them as pets and handled quite large spiders with no fear. When the father left home, she developed an acute fear of spiders, but could now more easily handle a 'daddy-long-legs', insects which in the past she had feared. The link to the lost daddy was clear from the insect imagery and the dreaded spider contained some other dreaded event and emotion associated with the loss of the father - perhaps his death, or embodying all the ambivalent feelings she felt towards him for having left her and the family. Phobias are often suggested by parents who impose their own fears and primitive symbols upon their children, just as they were imposed upon them by their own parents. This often is the reason for a fear of mice, snakes, or illogical situations, where it is the insecurity of the parent which is at the root of the child's fear, rather than any deep-rooted problem within the child.

Remedies to consider:

Argentum nit   For panicky phobic attacks, in the insecure child, aggravated by heat. There are claustrophobic anxieties with fear of being shut in an enclosed space. Also fear of heights.

Belladonna   The child is overactive and restless, the skin hot, red and dry, often with a slightly raised temperature. There are fears of nightmare-like threatening figures, faces, animals, monsters with impulses to run away, escape. He is frequently tearful and difficult to reassure.

Natrum mur   For the phobic child who lacks confidence and is never at ease in any social situation. Typically he fears being attacked, or he may be preoccupied with a fear of burglars.

EXCESSIVE POSSETTING

This is due to regurgitation of undigested food by the young baby, usually milk. It tends to occur where feeding has been overdone, too much food given too quickly, with faulty technique, usually by an inexperienced mother either at the breast or bottle.

It is best treated by prevention and allowing the child to suck more slowly, gently pacing the intake of food. Winding the child regularly on the shoulder every five to ten minutes during the feeds,is helpful, and then after the feed, either on the shoulder, or the baby held upright on the knee.

The condition is usually without significance and, as the mother gains experience and confidence, the problem tends to resolves spontaneously. If it should persist, the mother is advised to talk initially to her health visitor.

Remedies to consider:

Aethusa   Where the regurgitation is directly
                            related to sensitivity to cow's
                            milk.

Nux vom   For problems of colicky windy
                            pains with regurgitation and
                            irritability.

Pulsatilla   When symptoms are more
                            variable, the child tearful and
                            intolerant of heat.

PROJECTILE VOMITING

This usually occurs in the first 6 to 8 weeks of birth and mainly in male babies. It is of unknown cause, but due to Pyloric Stenosis or thickening of the muscular pyloric exit area of the stomach. It is only rarely found in females.

The main danger to the baby is dehydration and weight loss. It is completely cured by surgery. In a few cases it is due to simple vomiting with a mixture of undigested food and wind. If this more benign form of vomiting persists, it may also lead to weight loss, which in the young baby is always serious and may require admission to a specialised paediatric unit.

In some cases there may be a partial pyloric stenosis which may resolve spontaneously as the child matures, without the necessity for surgery as long as the child continues to thrive with a satisfactory weight gain. But whenever vomiting is persistent, it should be investigated, particularly if there is weight loss.

In most cases, vomiting of any kind is due to wind and indigestion, requiring simple common sense measures such as slowing the rate of feeding and winding the baby. Sometimes forceful vomiting may be associated with milk intolerance and with these babies, a soya formulation is indicated, and cures the problem.

Remedies to consider:

Aethusa Where the underlying problem is intolerance of cow's milk.

Carbo veg For the child who is sleepy, sluggish and weak, with associated problems of wind, colic and abdominal distention, usually from swallowing air when feeding, either at the breast or bottle.

Nux vomica For children who are constipated, irritable, with colicky pain, either before or after feeding. Sudden spasms of projectile vomiting may occur.

Zincum met The food is quickly vomited, without nausea or retching, the child weak with a tendency to loss of weight.

ROSACEA (Seborrhoeic skin rash)

A seborrhoeic skin condition which mainly involves the skin of the face, but especially the cheeks, with redness and an irritating rash of small isolated red spots which may become yellow and quite sore.

The condition is very similar to eczema and associated with an excessive oily or greasy discharge from the seborrhoeic skin glands within the pores. Usually the temperature remains normal. The skin area has a tendency to flaking and dryness. It may occasionally becomes infected, because of scratching.

The affected skin area should be cleansed with plain warm water during normal washing. The mother should not be tempted to apply any creams, as these will add to the greasy barrier already present. Because of an increase in the blood circulation, the rash often looks worse when the child is warm, for example the spots look darker, more intensely red when the baby has been sleeping on one side of the face.

There is no known cause, or satisfactory conventional treatment, although in some cases, hydrocortisone is prescribed. The condition usually cures spontaneously, although in a few cases, it becomes chronic. Homoeopathy is usually both safe and effective.

Remedies to consider:

Belladonna   When the skin is hot, dry and burning, the child restless and irritable.

Rhus tox   The skin condition is mild and irritating, the child wants to rub or scratch the area. All symptoms are aggravated by cold water or air and better for warmth.

Sulphur   The rash is discharging and dirty-looking. The child usually has an insatiable appetite and an offensive diarrhoea. All symptoms are worse from heat or washing.

Thuja   The child sweats profusely with an offensive oily sweat on covered parts and is full of contradictions. For example he is chilly, yet usually feels worse from the heat of the bed.

RUBELLA

Rubella or German Measles is an acute viral infection of children and adults. It is always a mild illness, with an incubation period of 14 to 21 days . The main symptoms are malaise with a brief flat pale diffuse rash resembling measles. Often the rash only lasts a few hours, accompanied by swollen and tender neck lymphatic glands, usually only present for a very short period.

The only significance of the infection is a high risk of foetal abnormality when it occurs in pregnancy.

It is now standard practise to vaccinate all children, both boys and girls, with the specific Rubella virus vaccine in the second year of life, and girls again between the age of 10 and 14. The illness itself does not usually need any specific treatment and tends to cure spontaneously.

An infected child should always be kept isolated from any pregnant members of the family, and also from an unvaccinated woman, who may be pregnant.

Remedies to consider:

Aconitum   A useful remedy for the early stages of rubella, when there is malaise, headache and painful neck lymphatic glands.

Belladonna   There is a sore throat, the child hot, sweating, with headache and the typical rash.

Rhus tox   There is a mild irritating pink measles-like transient rash, all symptoms better for warmth and fresh air with exercise.

Rubella nosode   The homoeopathic vaccine-equivalent, taken in a 30c potency dose to prevent or treat the infection.

Sulphur   For more drawn-out symptoms of fatigue, stomach discomfort with diarrhoea and an insatiable appetite. The skin is often infected and discharging.

RUNNING AWAY

A secure child rarely runs away from home, although he may explore areas increasingly distant from his home base as confidence and security grow. Insecurity is more likely to cause a child to run away, especially in a split one-parent or step-family, where the child is unhappy, depressed, confused, feels unwanted, and in need of attention. Occasionally running away is a sign of aggression and independence, again more common in a family in crisis or where it is split, the child emotionally damaged by events that have happened. Sometimes a child who runs away, takes the initiative because he feels that he is in control, and that the mother cannot leave him. But in most cases, the child who runs away does not really want to leave. He wants to be noticed, to feel valued, to know that he is important, loved by his parents and sometimes by his siblings. Running away signifies the need to be looked for and to be found. Anger, disapproval, or punishment, is preferable to feeling ignored and unwanted. When it is an isolated incident, the child often wants to provoke the mother to give him more attention and concern, to show love and caring for him more overtly. This sometimes occurs after the birth of a sibling, the child feeling he comes second after the new baby. But these problems can usually be dealt with by the mother giving the child more individual time for play and discussion. If the problem persists, with possible risks to the child, counselling help is often needed, but parents should always give as much individual time as is practicable. If it is an isolated occurrence, it should still be talked about but not given undue prominence. In an older child, physical bullying, sexual abuse, sometimes physical deprivation, may be underlying reasons.

Remedies to consider:

Argentum nit   The child is anxious, feels very insecure, running away to avoid a situation he feels unable to cope with, or because he needs attention and more reassurance. Running away is psychologically a way of obtaining it. The child is typically intolerant of heat.

Natrum mur   For a nervous insecure child or teenager, never at ease in a social situation and tending to avoid others. He is tearful and full of fears about the past or the future, needing more confidence and experience and to learn social skills with other children.

Nux vomica   For the irritable fractious child who is impulsive, lacking the ability to stop and think a situation through. He tends to be led by extremes of emotions, moving from tears to exasperation if he does not his get way.

Pulsatilla   The child lacks confidence, is fearful and easily tearful.

Silicea   For the small, puny, easily frightened child who runs away. He is often bullied or abused.

SEA SICKNESS

This can be a severe problem for a child, especially when anticipation of the sea crossing causes added emotions of excitement and fear. In a sensitive child, any excess emotion tends to exacerbate the problem - typically nausea and malaise - from disturbance of the balance centre of the inner ear caused by the rocking movements of the boat.

The psychological aspects of the problem are well known and fear, or lack of confidence add to the severity of any symptoms. Where the parents are quiet and not anxious, resting quietly if they feel nausea, or perhaps walking around if they are not affected by the movement, then the children are less likely to be so severely affected by the crossing.

If the child is susceptible to vomiting, it is best to keep him as quiet as possible and not to give him heavy fatty or greasy meals until land is in sight after a short crossing, or when he feels totally well and confident on a longer trip.

The condition tends to be aggravated by looking at an oscillating horizon, and most children are better for lying down and staying calm. Avoid reading, looking at the sea and heavy indigestible meals just before travelling. During the crossing, give the child plenty of fluids. Warm drinks are preferable to ice cold drinks or iced lollies.

Remedies to consider:

Cocculus   The child feels faint and sick or vomits. There is aversion to food or drink. The mouth and tongue has a metallic taste. All symptoms are worse for tobacco smoke and from cold air.

Kreosotum   The child has attacks of nausea with vomiting. He is usually thirsty and restless.

Nux vomica   The child is irritable with spasms of nausea and sickness, the stomach tender and distended. The tongue and mouth has a sour taste. A strong desire persists for food, especially for fried foods immediately after vomiting. He is worse for dry, cold air and better for damp warm conditions.

Petroleum   The child complains of a sharp taste on the tongue and in the mouth. After vomiting the child is very hungry, but has a strong aversion to fried foods, fats, or cabbage. All symptoms are worse from damp and better for warmth.

Tabacum   Sweating with weakness, pallor, tremor and shaking are the major symptoms indicating this very useful remedy.

SHYNESS

The shy child is usually uncomfortable and sensitive and needing help. Shyness is associated with a tendency to hold down emotions, often because they are feared and felt to be either dangerous, or unwelcome in the family, because emotions are not expressed and tolerated.

Shyness problems start early, with a tendency to withhold and to lack spontaneity, especially with adults, or with anyone new or strange, also in new situations.

A shy child holds back and is cautious as he sums up the situation, with unhealthy emotional attitudes, holding in feelings, needs and attitudes, especially in the presence of authority figures.

Shyness can be regarded as a compromise situation, expressing both anger and shame, a need for attention as well as shrinking from the limelight. Mild shyness is not important and usually disappears with maturity, but if severe and persistent, it should be discussed within the family, encouraging conversation and more spontaneity of expression of feelings.

The parents should also take a look at their own relationship, to see how open they are with each other and the children. They may also want to consider if they have been more strict for any reason with this particular child, why this happened and how to remedy it.

Remedies to consider:

Argentum nit For the phobic or panicky child who is intolerant of heat in any form, adding to his insecurity because he feels faint and fears losing control in public.

Gelsemium For the nervous shy child with mild shyness, easily nervous and frightened by any new situation and tending to avoid social contacts with other children. The social isolation tends to feed his fears and creates further loss of confidence.

Natrum mur For the rather weak anxious child, easily tearful, never comfortable in the company of others and often depressed. All of this leads to a child who is severely underfunctioning both socially and often intellectually for his age and ability.

Pulsatilla The child tends to be bright and creative, yet passive and attention seeking, feeling mortified, if in the limelight. He is easily tearful, with sudden mood changes, better for company and social contacts. Many of the problems are aggravated by heat. Lack of thirst is characteristic.

SLEEP PROBLEMS

For a variety of reasons, children frequently have problems with their sleep routine. Often there is a clear-cut physical reason with discomfort or pain, a raised temperature, the child unwell and unable to relax. Other causes include a room that is too hot, cold or noisy, or when the child is incubating one of the acute infections, such as measles. Most physical sleep problems improve when the underlying causes are removed and the child feels more relaxed. Emotional causes are a common reason for not sleeping, the child restless, unable to fall asleep because his mind is overactive. There may be excitement or fear about a coming event, a holiday, moving house, change of school, a friend coming to stay. If the child is depressed, the problem may be waking early, or sleeping lightly and waking throughout the night. Parents should try to ensure that bedtimes are a relaxed happy end to the day, where problems of anger or irritation towards the child are dispelled, and a fresh start made to the following day. Your health visitor will discuss a sleep management programme, which can be combined with homoeopathy.

SLEEP WALKING
This sometimes occurs in young children, although more common in the older child and teenager.It is associated with a very deep form of sleep and usually without significance. When it occurs nightly, it may be part of an emotional disturbance. It is not harmful to wake the child, and the child usually remembers nothing of the incident. If linked to other symptoms of insecurity, the child nervous, perhaps avoiding other children, give him more individual time, and encourage the child to talk about his main areas of fear or anxiety.

Remedies to consider:

Coffea The child is restless, his mind too active. He may also complain of awareness of his heart beating, stomach cramps and sweating.

Gelsemium For the anxious hysterical child, easily getting into an emotional state or panic at a visit or change of routine. The child is often tired and prefers to play alone.

Lycopodium For the fearful child who is over-excitable before a family trip or before a change of routine. The child is full of anticipatory anxieties, eventually falling into a restless sleep.

Natrum mur The child is anxious throughout the day. The problems at night are a continuation of this with fear of the dark, of dreaming, or being left alone in his room.

Pulsatilla For the anxious child, often depressed, tearful, sensitive to heat and mood changes. Sleep talking may occur.

PARENTAL SMOKING, RISKS FOR THE CHILD

Smoking is high risk during and after pregnancy. The child is affected by secondary (passive) smoking or inhalation of tobacco smoke in the home environment.

Particularly the sinuses, throat and bronchial tubes become irritated by the smoke, which causes congestion and thickening of the lining layers, leading to a cough with thick white or yellow mucus phlegm.

This problem is best approached by both parents stopping the habit at least several months before the child is conceived and it should be a major part of pre-conceptual planning and thinking by every caring couple.

The risks for the baby or child are considerable, and it may easily lead to permanent damage and chronic lung problems from an early age.

There is increased risk of bronchitis, asthma, and chest infections, also upper respiratory problems such as recurrent coughs and colds, sinus infection and sore throat.

The child is more vulnerable to infections of any type, especially when the mother smoked during pregnancy, or the child was born with a low birth weight.

Remedies to consider:

Arsenicum   The child is thin, constantly tired with a weak chest. Every cold goes to the chest with asthma, recurrent coughs, or bronchitis. Most symptoms are worse in the early night hours, the child waking worse from cold, with a cough, or asthma.

Bryonia   There is a chronic dry cough, worse for heat, movements or exercise.

Lycopodium   There is a right-sided chest weakness, with asthma or bronchitis, which may turn to pneumonia. All symptoms are worse in the late afternoon and early evening.

Phosphorus   For the thin chilly child with chest weakness and recurrent attacks of asthma.

Tabacum   For the chesty child with sensitivity to tobacco smoke which causes coughing, shortness of breath, bronchitis, or asthma.

SOILING

This is commonly in young children when there is an emotional crisis in the family and it is only rarely due to a physical cause.

Soiling tends to occur in a child who is lacking in confidence and unable to verbalise well. this is often because the family themselves do not use words easily and the child has been brought up in a closed situation where verbal communication and emotions are both kept tightly under a lid. It may follow when a sensitive child has been humiliated, particularly if this occurred in public.

The problem tends to recur and is different from an isolated 'accident' which occurs because of diarrhoea. Soiling is usually more severe than bed-wetting, which is much more common, and it can occur even in families which verbalise well.

Counselling may be needed for a recurrent problem, especially where the parents find talking about feelings to be difficult. Where the onset is clearly linked to an obvious psychological situation which may be threatening the child, such as a new pregnancy, a new baby, the death of a sibling, fear of going into hospital or starting a new school, then these can best be talked about within the security of the home.

If the problem persists it is worth discussing it with your local homoeopathic doctor, health visitor, or local teacher if the child is in school.

Remedies to consider:

Argentum nit   The child is fearful and phobic, the soiling aggravated by heat and emotion.

Arsenicum   There is a chilly diarrhoea, the child anxious, fussy and obsessional. All symptoms are worse after midnight.

Lycopodium   For the anxious child who reacts to all new situation with gassy indigestion and flatulence, or diarrhoea with soiling.

Natrum mur   The child lacks security, is a loner, fearful of all new situations and never at ease with others. The soiling may occur when a new baby arrives, the child regressing because of underlying insecurity.

Podophyllum   For problems of recurrent painless diarrhoea, aggravated by eating acid fruits. All symptoms are worse in the morning or when teething.

Pulsatilla   For the shy child, who is easily tearful. All symptoms are worse for heat.

SQUINTING

A squint when one eye has a tendency to 'wander' is quite normal in a young baby for the first three months, as there is immaturity of the eye controlling muscles and lack of co-ordination.

The condition usually clears spontaneously without any treatment being necessary as the child matures. If it persists after the age of 3 months, it should be reported to the doctor or health visitor for monitoring and possible treatment.

Many improve with simple 'patching' or covering of the strong eye with a pad, encouraging the 'lazy' eye to work more. If it still persists, surgery may be needed to shorten or adjust the length of the specific optical muscles responsible for eye co-ordination.

The results from surgery are usually satisfactory, and the operation is recommended when the condition does not respond to simple measures such as 'patching' combined with homoeopathy.

Remedies to consider:

Gelsemium There is disturbed visual co-ordination because of weakness of one group of eye muscle.There may be blurring or visual discomfort when accommodating to different visual objects. One pupil may be more dilated than the other. The child is usually passive, nervous and fearful. He lacks confidence with other children and with adults outside the immediate family.

Ruta The eye tends to give a lot of aching discomfort, especially after reading or any form of close work. The eye strain tends to be aggravated by cold or damp, also from poor light conditions.

SPEECH PROBLEMS

Stammering is usually due to an underlying psychological problem, the child too tense and unsure of himself. Usually only certain sounds and letters are stammered, lisped or slurred, the particular sound having become synonymous with the underlying emotional difficulty.

In some cases, the child has been brought up too strictly, made to be prematurely clean and neat because of parental intolerance and insecurity, with little room for him to express any natural aggression or rebellion. He is often quiet, too well behaved and compliant, only able to express more defiant feelings in this way. With other children, who are not really wanted and feel rejected, the stammer becoming a way of getting individual attention and time.

Often the problem is best dealt with by family therapy and homoeopathy, looking at the underlying emotional issues, and the extent of any rigidity or unreasonable controls within the family unit, trying to improve health and confidence, with greater tolerance and more open communication of ideas and feelings.

Lisping is a milder slurring speech defect of the young. It usually clears completely with the help of a speech therapist as the child grows and matures. Orthodox medication is of no value in the condition and only rarely is surgery, indicated to free the tongue, rarely occurring as tongue-tie. Most cases improve with homoeopathy, but the results are even better, if the clarity of speech and confidence are also built up by regular visits to an experienced Speech Therapist.

Remedies to consider:

Causticum   The tongue seems slow to move. Co-ordination is poorly established, as if the child is tongue-tied.

Natrum mur   For the anxious insecure child who is never verbally at ease in any new or social situation.

Nux vomica   The child is irritable and often aggressive, with a short-fuse disposition.

Phosphorus   For the nervous thin child who constantly needs reassurance, is anticipating disapproval or criticism and is terrified of this.

Pulsatilla   For varied speech problems, for example a lisp, in a shy, easily tearful passive child who lacks confidence.

Sulphur   Indicated for more chronic problems, usually in an untidy overweight child, the lisp worse in the morning, also from heat and after bathing.

STINGS

The usual sting is from an insect bite, but it may also originate from plants, such as a stinging nettle, or one that provokes a strong allergic response. But in most cases a sting is caused by a wasp, bee, midge, fly, mosquito or hornet.

The cause is less important in homoeopathy than the type of reaction that occurs on the skin. Always completely remove the sting if it is still present in the skin and soothe the area with a healing cream such as Calendula.

Reassure the child. If the parents panic, the child often becomes hysterical and highly emotional, greatly increasing the physiological as well as emotional response.

Use a natural insect repellent, such as Citronella. If the child is prone to insect bites, and reacts severely, or is frightened of being stung, use Apis before the child goes into a country area.

If you are on holiday, in an area where a particular type of midge or fly is causing a painful sting, as sometimes occurs in hot humid conditions, consult a homoeopathic pharmacist for a specific remedy for the particular insect involved.

Remedies to consider:

Apis   The sting is red, swollen, angry looking and very tender. The child is usually restless, fearful and anxious.

Ledum   The sting is painful but cold, paradoxically better for a cold compress, but aggravated by heat.

Rhus tox   For mild red irritating stings, better for local warmth and movement, worse for damp or cold of any kind.

Ruta   The sting feels bruised, sore and painful, the child faint or weak. All symptoms are aggravated by damp or cold.

Urtica   The sting area is swollen with stinging itchy discomfort.

STYES

These are caused by a local infection of one of the hair follicles of the eye lash, often associated with rubbing the eye. This often causes a secondary infection from bacteria present on the skin of the fingers.

The underlying problem is usually due to a too high intake of sugars in the diet - such as sweets, ice cream, cakes, chocolate. These cause raised blood sugar levels and as a result, a rich environment where bacteria are able to flourish. One of their favourite areas, is the eye hair follicle because it provides a naturally warm and moist environment for them to proliferate. Styes are often recurrent.

Craving for sweet foods is often associated with an emotional disturbance, for example, feelings of deprivation, and the need for sugars is a substitute for affection.

The child should be encouraged not to rub his eye, the fingers kept clean, and nails clipped. If rubbing his eye is a symptom of tension and insecurity, the underlying causes should be looked for and discussed with the child.

Whenever there is a problem of any form of recurrent infection which does not clear up, always carefully examine the diet of the child to see if it is lacking and a cause for lowered vitality and resistance. Also consider a possible underlying emotional cause for the problem.

Remedies to consider:

Antimonium crud For an acute painful stye with a thick yellow discharge of pus.

Hepar sulph A useful remedy for styes which tend to recur, the child chilly and irritable and all symptoms worse from draughts of cold air.

Pulsatilla A remedy for recurrent variable stye problems, the child shy and sensitive, easily tearful and often rubbing the affected eye because of anxiety and tension, or after crying. The problem is aggravated by heat in any form and is better for a local cool compress. The child usually has a high dietary sugar intake which further aggravates the problem.

Silicea For chronic stye problems which discharge pus. The child is weak, sweats on exposed surfaces of his body and lacks confidence and drive.

SUNBURN

This may be a problem for young children when they have been exposed for long periods to the sun at the beginning of a holiday without adequate protection. Remember to choose carefully a barrier cream which protects the child from both alpha and beta rays of the sun, not just the latter as both are important causes of sunburn.

The condition is best treated by prevention, not allowing children on the beach or in direct sun at mid-day. They should always be kept reasonably covered with a top shirt and hat when in direct heat and mainly allowed to play in the sun in the morning or late afternoon, keeping exposure minimal for the first few days until they have a tan and some resistance to the direct sun. In young babies this is especially important, but also with any small child, as skin burns can be very unpleasant and often deep, requiring admission to a special burns unit and in some cases a skin graft.

If sunburn has occurred, keep the child cool and in the shade, but not allowing him to become chilled. Ensure that the child does not become dehydrated by offering plenty of fluids. In most cases, sunburn is now treated by exposing the area affected to the air rather than by covering them with a dressing as in the past, but this does depend on the extent of the sunburn.

If in doubt get advice from your local doctor or casualty officer at the hospital. Calendula cream locally helps keep the area cool and more comfortable, but it is not recommended for very extensive or deep burns which are best treated in a paediatric special burns unit.

Remedies to consider:

Apis

There is stinging burning pain, with swelling of the area affected by the sunburn.

Belladonna

The area is burning hot, tender and swollen, worse for local heat of any kind, the child restless and anxious. The temperature may be raised because of the burn.

Calendula

A useful healing remedy, applied as a cream to the burn area, or taken internally by mouth in the 6c potency.

Cantharis

For burning irritating sunburn problems, the area smarting and raw. Symptoms are relieved by a local cold compress, but worse for touching the affected area and for further exposure to heat in any form.

Rhus tox

The area of burn feels itchy, red and uncomfortable, often slightly swollen or thickened, but better for a warm compress and for movement. All symptoms are aggravated by cold in any form.

Sol

A useful remedy for mild sunburn reactions.

SWALLOWED OBJECTS

These are best removed by holding a small child upside down and using gentle persuasion to encourage him to cough up and regurgitate the swallowed item. The child should be reassured, the parents staying calm, in this way relaxing him, and encouraging its removal without provoking undue pain or stress.

If the swallowed object is toxic, for example:- the mother's contraceptive 'pill', carbon paper, or cold cream, or suspected to be so, it is best to take the child immediately to hospital for an opinion. Most items are usually small, round and firm, and their removal is easy. If it has passed through the stomach into the intestine, it cannot be removed by regurgitation, and its passage and eventual excretion in the stools, may require monitoring using x-ray and modern scan techniques.

The healthy toddler, exploring his environment, is likely to place any brightly coloured object into his mouth as part of his natural curiosity and development. For this reason, medication belonging to the parents, should be kept locked away, out of reach and danger. At the same time, the child should be taught not to put unknown bright shining objects into his mouth. Berries and seeds are often potentially toxic and a particular danger.

Remedies to consider:

Arnica   This is useful to reduce swelling and bruising within the oesophagus as the result of irritation and minor damage caused by what has been mouthed and swallowed.

Calcarea   The child is passive, chilly and with obsessional tendencies.

Chamomilla   Useful where objects are placed in the mouth to relieve teething pain or discomfort.

Staphisagria   For discomfort due to oesophageal irritation or damage.

TANTRUMS

Temper tantrums are common at some time with every child. They are usually an expression of rage and frustration at being held in check, when the child's natural instinct is to explore, to mouth and to touch, often to throw away or to break his toys into pieces.

A tantrum may be due to hunger, pain, colic, or not being able to understand or co-ordinate a movement that the child has a desire to gratify immediately. For a young child, any delay seems an obstacle to his need for instant satisfaction. He may throw a tantrum to express anger, particularly trying to influence the mother and gain her attention. Usually this kind of behaviour lessens by the age of three.

If a tantrum occurs in an older child, the mother should remain calm and relaxed, talking to the child, trying to persuade him to behave a little more reasonably. With a younger child, a tantrum is often best ignored. If a tantrum relates to physical pain, (for example during teething, because of hay fever or abdominal colic), this must be diagnosed, the cause found and treated.
It does not help to shout during a tantrum or to smack the child. This usually encourages more shouting, and smacking is usually only a temporary release for the mother, but does not resolve the underlying problem. Physical punishment may lead to depression and resentment, or the child bullying in later years. Always ascertain the cause of the tantrum without delay and then deal with the problem at this level. Once the child understands that there is a reason for refusal to give in to his demands, if the mother stays calm, the child usually responds to the explanations and attention given.

Remedies to consider:

Chamomilla   For a restless, complaining and often whining irritable child who wants to be held and reassured all the time. As soon as he is put down, either to sleep or to walk, he has a tantrum expressing outrage and resentment at no longer having continual attention. The child is usually constantly thirsty and worse for all forms of heat.

Nux vomica   For an irritable child with frequent problems of stomach cramp with wind and colicky pains. The child is usually worse on a hot day and better when the day is both cool and damp. Constipation is a very common problem.

Tarentula   For the most violent forms of temper tantrums, the child often changeable and very moody. He is usually sensitive to music which tends to calm him. The child prefers to be alone, and dislikes company.

TEETHING PROBLEMS

All children experience some pain and discomfort, becoming more irritable when the milk teeth emerge and their gums hurt. Salivation and dribbling increases, and children want to put something firm in their mouths to try to find comfort. They are naturally more fretful at this time, find sleep difficult, waking with pain, crying and often uninterested in food. Teething happens from about the age of four months, the child irritable, with minimal intermittent discomfort, but not normally ill or physically unwell. If symptoms continue, these may need to be reassessed, and not just assumed to be due to 'teething'. Always give reassurance and comfort to the child, and explain what is happening and the reason why discomfort is occurring.

TEETH GRINDING

When the teeth are ground together during sleep, it is often a symptom of underlying tension and anxiety. If allowed to continue without treatment, it may in the long term harm the dental shape and bite. Giving the child more time, looking in detail at the child's temperament, levels of achievement and confidence, abilities for self-expression, control over anger and aggression, are some of the areas which may be helpful to discuss. Rarely there is a physical cause, for example threadworm, or there has been brain damage. Such causes are however uncommon and most cases are psychological in origin. Specialised counselling may be required for a time if the problem does not improve with parental discussion combined with the homoeopathic approach.

Remedies to consider:

Belladonna

The child is restless and anxious, the temperature slightly elevated, his face red, burning and swollen. All symptoms are aggravated by heat.

Chamomilla

For teething problems where the child is complaining, miserable, irritable and restless, wanting to be constantly held and reassured. He cries with rage and resentment when put down, but feels better for warm drinks and warm applications to any tender areas.

Cina

The child tends to be large and overweight with problems of teeth grinding and irritability. Hunger is constant, with constipation and small pale stools. Irritation of the nose and anal area is common.

Hepar sulph

The child is intensely irritable, the gums swollen, sore and painful to touch. All symptoms are better for warmth and moist damp conditions and covering or wrapping the head.

Nux vomica

The child is irritable, complaining of sudden spasms of toothache, aggravated by cold air.

THROAT PROBLEMS

Acute sore throat is one of the most common of all childhood problems. It can occur at any age and may be accompanied by a rise in temperature, painful throat, tenderness on swallowing and painful lymphatic glands in the neck area. The child feels unwell, is uninterested in food, lethargic, tearful, whining and demanding more attention. Where the cause is viral rather than bacterial, the response to repeated courses of antibiotics is often less than positive, tending to deplete vitality reserves, and to dampen down the natural immune defence system of the body. The child should be kept cool with plenty of fluids and honey drinks with lemon until the temperature falls. It is best not to give the child solid foods when there is a raised temperature, but clear soups and other drinks, may be given liberally at this time, and he should be allowed to suck ice lollies.

LARYNGITIS

Inflammation of the larynx is common in childhood and usually manifests as a sore throat with hoarseness, sometimes loss of the voice or it varies in pitch with lack of control of sounds created, speech sometimes reduced to a whisper. It often occurs quickly in a young child, with a sore throat and enlarged tender neck glands. It is important to rest the voice as much as possible, especially from excessive talking, excitable speech, or any form of strain or shouting. A steam inhalation often relieves the condition. The condition is usually short-lived, clearing within a few days. Only rarely does it become chronic, and more likely in an older child. If recurrent a paediatric opinion should be sought.

Remedies to consider:

Antimonium crud For acute throat conditions with a thick yellow or creamy catarrhal discharge.The child is irritable, symptoms worse in the evening and improved by warm moist air.

Baryta carb The throat is acutely inflamed, swallowing painful, tonsils and neck glands enlarged and tender.

Belladonna For very acute throat infections, the area red raw, the temperature elevated and the child restless.

Causticum A very useful remedy for laryngitis. The voice is low or hoarse, often with a dry cough.

Hepar sulph The throat is painful and sore with stitch-like sharp pains, worse on swallowing. The temperature is elevated, the child irritable.

Lachesis For left-sided throat infections, the area purplish-blue and very tender. Symptoms are aggravated by swallowing or the least touch.

Pyrogenium The temperature of the child is high with a hot, red, dry throat. Talking and swallowing difficult.

Sulphur For recurrent throat problems.

THRUSH

The common fungal infection of children due to the yeast organism Candida albicans. It usually affects either the mouth or vagina, with a milky-white discharge, looking like curds of milk which may bleed and leave a raw-looking area underneath. They may occur on the tongue, gums and beneath the cheek areas of the young child and also within the vaginal area. Thrush is always aggravated by moisture and warmth. Nappies should be changed frequently, or disposed of altogether during the period of infection, leaving the genital area exposed to the air as far as is practicable.

Nappies should be rinsed well of all detergent residues, as this may further aggravate the condition. In addition to the homoeopathic remedies recommended, the area affected can be carefully dabbed with 1% Potassium Permanganate or 1% Gentian Violet. to help destroy the yeast organisms.

About 80% of nappy area infections are fungal in origin. It can sometimes spread to the mother, causing sore nipples and an itchy breast. Every mother should examine the inside of her child's mouth to check for the white fungal infected patches, which can't be wiped off and stay attached to the mucosa. The most likely cause is alteration of the normal flora(bacterial inhabitants) of the intestinal tract after a course of antibiotics. Giving the child natural yogurt helps to re-colonise the bowel flora and to lessen the thrush problem.

Remedies to consider:

Antimonium crud   The child is irritable, the affected area dry, often cracked, bleeding easily and with a white slimy discharge. Symptoms tend to be worse in the evening and are aggravated by heat or contact with water.

Natrum mur   The child is without energy, tearful, anxious, restless, avoiding other children. The lower lip tends to crack, also the corners of the mouth. There is a thin white mucus discharge, the thrush area dry and irritated.

Rhus tox   The area is red, raised and irritating, worse for cold water or cold air, but improved by warmth.

THUMB SUCKING

This is a comfort habit, which has usually continued from early infancy. The thumb comes to symbolise reassurance and continuity, which is there on demand, and cannot be taken away.

The underlying motivation for the habit, is often a compelling need for oral (mouth) satisfaction and security, at a time when he feels threatened in some way.

The threat may not be immediately obvious, as often any psychological damage occurred in the past and dates back to a key stage of psychological development. At this time the child may have felt particularly frightened, deprived, or threatened. A typical example, is where weaning was carried out too early, or in a precipitant way. In this instance, the thumb comes to symbolise the comfort, security and closeness of the lost early breast-relationship.

It is a mistake to suddenly try to stop or deprive the child of any habit that is needed for reassurance and reasons of personal security. The parents can best help by reassuring the child, but also by encouraging him to share and talk about his feelings and not to be afraid of them.

Remedies to consider:

Nux vomica

For the immature, often irritable child who directs all emotional problems to his mouth or intestine (which is the reason for his frequent problems of indigestion and colicky pains when under pressure emotionally). He tends to be too intense and to take on the problems of others. He is always in an emotional mood or state at the wrongs of others and the world about him. At the same time the child often fails to perceive the quality of his own caring and understanding of others. Much of the tension is centred around the immediate family. The thumb sucking is an infantile means of escape from what is felt to be a critical outside world (usually the family).

Pulsatilla

Indicated for the insecure child who needs constant reassurance and deals with emotional problems by using the mouth as a comfort agency. He quickly feels that others are criticising or making fun of him, and often becomes angry or tearful, which undermines emotional growth. The child only rarely says what he really means and feels.

TONSILLITIS

The tonsils, or lymphatic organs within the throat, act as a first line of resistance, by localising infections to the tonsillar area and acting to prevent its spread to the deeper organs. They act like sentry guards for the body in an area where infection is common and bacteria multiply easily.

The condition may be acute or chronic, sometimes lasting as a mild irritating illness over a period of weeks or months before finally clearing. Repeated doses of antibiotics are often ineffective, or only helpful for a very short time. Recurrent tonsillitis is a common problem, because the attacks last for 7 to 10 days, often recurring again, as soon as the child returns to school.

An affected child may quite easily be away from school for a major part of every term with a throat infection, raised temperature, feeling unwell, exhausted and uninterested in food, pale, and complaining. A constitutional, or nosode homoeopathic remedy, is usually required to improve the innate resistance and constitutional make-up of the child. This has often been impoverished by repeated courses of orthodox medication or as a reaction to vaccination.

Most cases respond well to homoeopathy without reducing the resistance and vitality of the child. In a few cases where the tonsils are large and chronically infected, surgery may be necessary, but it should be avoided if at all possible. The tonsils become naturally smaller as the child matures, and usually a less acute problem. As the overall vitality of the child improves, so too does the health of the tonsils.

Remedies to consider:

Antimonium crud The throat is sore, the tonsils large, infected and inflamed, the voice husky and croaky from an associated laryngitis. The child is irritable and complaining, worse in the evening from heat.

Baryta carb The throat is extremely sore with sharp stitch-like pains, the neck glands enlarged and tender. The child is anxious, tearful, lacking in confidence, better for fresh air.

Belladonna For acute tonsillitis, the throat raw, tender on swallowing, the face red, dry and hot from the high temperature.

Hepar sulph For recurrent attacks of tonsillar infection, the throat sore with sharp pains. The child is irritable, worse from cold air.

Lachesis The throat is inflamed, dark purplish-red, worse on the left side. The child is restless and anxious, all symptoms aggravated by touching the throat or neck.

Lycopodium For right-sided tonsillar infections, the pain and discomfort worse in the late afternoon or early evening.

UNDESCENDED TESTICLE

A condition where usually one testicle remains in the abdominal cavity without descending into the testicle pouch.

The male testicle is usually fixed in the scrotum at birth, although in some boys, the testicle is mobile and when touched, will retract back into the abdomen, where it first developed. The condition usually corrects itself spontaneously in the early years, without any specific treatment and the testicle becomes firmly fixed within the scrotum, as the residual channel linking it to the abdomen closes up.

It is important to correct a persistent undescended testicle for future health, because there is a slight risk of malignancy, or the testicle may not function well if left undescended. Where it does not descend spontaneously or with the help of a homoeopathic remedy, then surgery is indicated to ensure that the testicle is correctly positioned.

Opinions vary on the best time for an operation, but many surgeons now feel that it should be done early, from one to two years of age.

In many areas, undescended testicle is now routinely screened for at the age of one year, by either the health visitor or general practitioner.

Remedies to consider:

Aurum met The testicle is often tender, painful or swollen, the child tending to be irritable or depressed.

Pulsatilla The child is typically fair, often passive and shy and quickly moved to tears or other emotions. He is quite intolerant of heat in all forms and is only comfortable in the fresh air and for movement.

URTICARIA

An allergic irritating skin reaction, resembling nettle rash, with thickening, redness, blister formation, or a raised white or red area, which may ooze a clear straw-coloured fluid. In sensitive individuals, it may be caused by intolerance to a particular food, such as strawberries, dairy products, colourants, washing powders. Other causes are:- allergy to feathers, animal hair, chocolate, oranges, tomatoes, pollen, certain plants, also house-dust.

Rarely a severe urticaria reaction occurs in the throat, (angioneurotic oedema), the child in a panic and unable to breath because the lips, throat and larynx swell rapidly. Immediate hospitalisation and taking the child to casualty is recommended. Such reactions are rare, but they may occur after an acute sensitivity reaction to an insect sting or certain medications.

Children may sometimes react very severely to just one tablet of children's aspirin. It is now officially banned for all children under the age of 12 years of age because of the possible risk of Reye's syndrome - an acute illness with encephalitis, fever, vomiting, progressive coma and fits.

The response to homoeopathy is safe, usually rapid and effective.

Remedies to consider:

Apis
The skin is pink, swollen and irritating, or painful and stinging. The child is typically anxious and restless. All symptoms are aggravated by any form of heat.

House dust
For house-dust mite sensitivity reactions, the skin red, blotchy, swollen and intensely irritating.

Rhus tox
The skin is raised, red or pink, with blisters, the whole area very sensitive and irritated, but better for the local application of warmth and better for fresh air and movement.

Urtica
There is a burning stinging urticaria, which looks and feels as if the child has been in contact with stinging nettles. Blister formation may occur, which discharges a clear fluid.

VACCINATION ALTERNATIVES

Many parents are totally in favour of the official policies of routine vaccination without question. Others are more sceptical of routine prophylactic immunisation for their child and consider that the risks may outweigh the advantages, i.e. that the child's health and natural immunity may suffer or be permanently damaged.

In some cases the child may not be suitable for immunisation because of a past or family history of neurological symptoms, especially fits which greatly add to the risks of brain damage, especially after immunisation for whooping cough.

For such children, or where the parents have a rooted objection to the whole concept of injecting a healthy child with a live virus or viral extract, then homoeopathy offers a no-risk alternative.

These should be discussed with your homoeopathic doctor and are not recommended for self-treatment.

Remedies to consider:

The specific nosodes (vaccination-equivalents)

of:-   Chickenpox
        Diphtheria
        German measles
        Measles
        Mumps
        Tuberculosis
        Whooping cough

VAGINA - FOREIGN BODY

Self exploration of every body orifice is normal for all children and part of growth and the normal learning process. Children often insert small round objects, such as beads, into their orifices, and the vagina is often used as a receptacle during these attempts to explore and discover more about the body, its boundaries and how it works.

In most cases no harm occurs and it is only when the child pushes something into the vagina that remains there and causes an infection that it is noticed. Usually the first symptom is a white or yellow discharge which may be unpleasant smelling and the vulva area becomes red or tender.

If bleeding occurs from the child using a sharp object, the upper vaginal area may become infected from urinary or faecal organism causing discomfort on passing urine.

If a foreign body is present it must be removed, preferably by the mother in the bath tub, or if this cannot be done, the child should be taken to her local doctor for advice.

Self-exploration of the vagina with the finger is normal and should be ignored. The child should never be blamed or made to feel guilty in any way.

Remedies to consider:

Antimonium crud   The vaginal area is tender inflamed, red, irritated and has developed an infection with a thick offensive creamy-yellow discharge. The child is often either tearful or irritable.

Apis   The area is red, swollen and painful, very sensitive to touch, the child restless and anxious, aggravated by any form of heat.

Belladonna   There is an intense burning and irritating vaginal reaction, with discharge and restlessness, the child intolerant of heat.

Calendula   A useful general remedy to promote healing, either applied locally to the vaginal area as a cream, or taken by mouth.

Hepar sulph   There are sharp vaginal pains and irritation because of an infection with a thin offensive discharge. The child is usually intensely peevish and irritable.

Rhus tox   The vaginal area is red and inflamed, very tender to touch, better for warm baths to the area, also improved by movement, but aggravated by cold in any form.

VAGINITIS

Infection of the vaginal mucosa or lining cellular layer, is common in children. The cause is often unknown, although most cases are thought to due to bacterial infection, from contamination by faeces, or due to a yeast (or Candida) infection. Vaginitis may also be associated with a urinary infection. The commonest symptoms are itchy stinging vaginal discomfort, and a discharge (leucorrhea), which may be clear, white, or thick, depending upon the type of infection. If there is a yeast infection, the discharge may have a strong or slightly fishy odour.

Most cases clear spontaneously with normal hygiene procedures i.e. keeping the area clean and soaped, and not leaving wet soiled nappies on for long periods, possibly removing them altogether until the infection clears, exposing the vulval area to the air as much as possible and keeping it dry. Talcum powder is not recommended. It is not sterile and may occasionally cause infection. When cleaning the child, wipe the anal area away from the vagina and never towards it. After urination, little girls should be taught to wipe themselves dry, to prevent contact of the delicate vaginal skin area with residual drops of stale urine. Tight clothing should be avoided in the pelvic area, and cotton pants are recommended. Bubble bath preparations should not be used for young children.

Recurrent unexplained vaginitis may possibly occur when the child is the victim of sexual interference or abuse. Any abnormal marks, bruising of the thigh or genital area, vaginal soreness or bleeding, using sexual words beyond the child's age, suggests this possibility.

Remedies to consider:-

Calendula For mild cases, the remedy helps to encourage healing.

Kali bich The vaginitis is mild, the discharge thick and yellow with burning irritation. The discharge is worse in the early hours, between 4.00 and 5.00am, aggravated by any form of heat.

Pulsatilla For mild variable symptoms, the discharge white or yellow, at times thick and offensive. It may be clear and fluid with little odour. The child is usually fair, passive and subject to mood swings, but especially to tears. All symptoms are aggravated by heat.

Silicea There is an acute infection with a thick offensive yellow pus discharge. The child is often thin and underweight, sweats profusely and she usually lacks confidence.

Sulphur For chronic vaginitis, the discharge thick and offensive, the surrounding skin red and inflamed. All symptoms are worse for heat and for contact with water.

VOMITING

Bringing up the contents of the stomach is common, and usually has a simple cause, provided it is not recurrent, or the child is losing weight. In most cases it occurs because of an infection, or where one is being incubated, for example, measles or chickenpox. The problem may also occur after swallowing a foreign body, for example a medication belonging to one of the parents, which the child assumed to be sweets. Swallowing too much food too quickly is another common non-infective cause of the problem. In a sensitive child, there is often an emotional cause, usually from excitement anxiety relating to a new school, anticipation of an outing or holiday. It also occurs from travelling, or when there has been a family emotional upset of some kind.

Repeated vomiting is really the only major cause for possible concern, especially when it occurs in young babies who are vulnerable to fluid loss and dehydration. Always ensure that a young child takes plenty of fluids, and these are best given after vomiting has occurred. If the baby repeatedly vomits more than twice a day, it should be reported to the doctor or health visitor and the cause ascertained. If the vomiting is not just a gentle evacuation of the stomach contents, but shoots out, as if from a cannon or water hose, then this should also be reported, especially if it occurs in a young baby. Other cases where vomiting should be discussed with the doctor or health visitor are:- if associated with diarrhoea, the child is obviously ill, has a temperature, is losing weight, when pain is associated with the vomiting, also when vomiting occurs after a head injury.

Remedies to consider:

Natrum mur   The vomiting is of psychological origin, the child fearful and lacking confidence. Vomiting is a symptom of fear of rejection, or anxiety about closeness, innovation and change. Tearful sad mood changes are common, the child thin and lacking energy.

Nux vomica   Vomiting is associated with painful spasms of indigestion pain, in an irritable child who has poor controls, and a short-fuse disposition. Constipation is usually another problem.

Pulsatilla   For the fair, rather shy passive child, who over-indulges in starchy carbohydrate foods which causes a gassy indigestion, wind and flatulence, often with a variable diarrhoea. There is a tearful disposition and swings of mood, from extremes of tears and sadness to laughter the next minute and just as quickly another shift of mood. All symptoms are worse for heat of any kind.

WHOOPING COUGH

One of the most dangerous acute infections of childhood, and especially a risk for the young baby, less so for an older child who is fit and healthy. The incubation period of Pertussis or whooping cough is 8-12 days and during this time the child is often restless and slightly unwell. The first sign is usually sudden and unexpected with the typical whoop after paroxysmal (continual) coughing, the whoop due to air being forced into the lungs through the narrowed larynx which is in spasm.

In some cases, the typical whoop does not develop, especially in very young children or babies, and the main symptom is severe and repetitive bouts of coughing, the child ill and listless, the cheeks often grey or mauve from cyanosis and lack of oxygen.

In most cases the illness is benign and there are few risks, the condition becoming self-limiting and slowly clearing up over a few weeks. The main danger is to the child under six months of age when frequency of coughing leads to exhaustion, dehydration and complete lack of energy and vitality. The major complication is a middle ear infection (otitis media) or pneumonia. Whooping cough is highly infectious and during the whoop phase the child should be kept away from other children.

The exact risks from the disease are hard to assess. During the 1978 epidemic only 12 deaths were notified in the U.K., although the true mortality from the disease may have been higher. It is advisable to keep the child reassured and relaxed, giving plenty of fluids, especially to a young child, after coughing or vomiting.

Remedies to consider:

Bryonia   Useful in late or convalescent cases, with a dry irritating cough, producing a clear or white phlegm.

Drosera   There are paroxysms of a most irritating dry cough followed by the characteristic whoop at the end of the coughing spasm, as the child gasps for air. The cough is worse for lying down and tends to occur in the early night hours.

Magnesium phos   Another useful remedy for dry, spasmodic bouts of coughing, all symptoms aggravated by lying down and at night. A warm room tends to improve the coughing.

Passiflora   Useful for spasm, the child restless and unable to sleep.

Pertusssin   The specific nosode or vaccination-equivalent. It is usually indicated at some time during the illness. It can be used to help prevent attacks, and to stimulate resistance against further infection and attacks.

Sulphur   For persistent cough, with a yellow or green offensive phlegm, worse in the mornings.

185

WILFUL AND DEFIANT BEHAVIOUR

Where the temperament of a child is strong, leading to self-willed determined independent aggression, he may pose a challenge for the parents. Often the problems are transient, arising at a time when the child feels insecure and not loved, for example after the birth of a younger brother or sister. There may be a variety of other reasons, including:- an enforced separation from the home, a family illness, an accident, or after an illness or an operation.

In all cases it is important for both parents to try to look at the causes when the wilful behaviour first began and why. There may have been an early separation from the mother which affected the child emotionally, he may be adopted, or experienced separation anxiety when just a few weeks old - perhaps because of an illness of either the child or the mother. It may also be associated with bullying. If linked to the birth of a sibling, the father also needs to help, making him feel loved and wanted, both parents demonstrating that he has an important role to play and an example to set. The child may become depressed, as part of feeling insecure, the wilful behaviour reflecting a need for more individual attention.

If the parents find this difficult, their health visitor may recommend some limited counselling for the child. At all times try not to be tense, irritable, rejecting and unfair with the child, as this is likely to lead to more problems.

Remedies to consider:

Chamomilla For the impatient demanding irritable child, who wants to be held constantly and when he does not have his way, or is put down to sleep or to play, has a tantrum of screaming rage with kicking and stamping. Behaviour is worse when teething and from heat.

Lycopodium The child is less aggressive than the above remedy, but he cannot be reasoned with. This is partly because he finds listening and concentration difficult, as he is always elsewhere, usually thinking ahead. As a result he is accident-prone and wilful because he quickly forgets what he has been told not to do. Basically he lacks confidence and is insecure.

Natrum mur For the fearful, insecure child who at times becomes irritable, flying into a rage when frustrated, often over a minor incident. Mood swings are common, and when he is not irritable and determined to have his way, he is tearful and sad.

Nux vomica For the irritable, short-fuse, aggressive, wilful, determined child.

WORMS

THREADWORM

This is a common problem affecting both the parents and children. For this reason, often the whole family requires treatment. The tiny threadworm lives in the anal region and is transported back to the mouth and intestinal tract (to renew its life cycle) by anal scratchings under the finger nails. To prevent re-infection, it is essential to keep the child's nails cut very short. Symptoms are itchy discomfort in the anal region, worse at night, nose scratching or picking, sleep disturbances and nightmares. The tiny parasites, like fine threads of wool, can be clearly seen in the anal region and on the stool.

ROUNDWORM

Roundworm infection is a major cause of blindness in childhood. It is increasingly recognized as a common cause of retinal damage and other illnesses of children. The most important source is from the roundworm of the dog, or Toxocara canis. The highly resistant eggs of an infected puppy or bitch survive in the soil for months, even years. In the UK about 2% of the population have the specific antibody, indicating infection at some time. The main risk is to young children playing in parks or on any area of soil contaminated by dog excrement. Human infection occurs from ingesting the eggs from contaminated fingers. The larvae, hatch out of the eggs, and travel to the liver, retina, muscles, and nervous system. Symptoms include, restlessness malaise, cough, throat infections, nausea, abdominal discomfort and nausea.

Remedies to consider:

Antimonium crud   For acute problems of pain and infection, the child irritable, with indigestion as shown by a white coating on the tongue. There is often a mixture of diarrhoea and constipation with anal itching.

Calcarea   The child is usually pale, bloated, passive and chilly with a sour diarrhoea and lack of energy.

Cina   The child is irritable overweight, pink-faced and always hungry. The nose itches, the umbilicus area is sore with a twisting discomfort and feeling irritable. The stools are small and pale, the anal area itchy. Vomiting occurs after eating, or there is diarrhoea after food.

Mercurius   The child is weak and tired, bathed in perspiration. The stool is slimy and uncomfortable, the stomach also painful. All symptoms tend to be worse at night and for heat or cold.

Pulsatilla   All symptoms are variable, the child shy and tearful, with marked mood swings, aggravated by heat. He is intolerant of fatty or fried food, but feels better for fresh air.

INDEX

HOMOEOPATHY

Understanding Homoeopathy (£6.95)

The revised second edition of this comprehensive book explains in clear, simple terms the basic principles of homoeopathy, which can be readily understood by the beginner. The author outlines the approach, indications, and choice of remedies for the common health problems of the family.

Talking About Homoeopathy (£4.95)

An invaluable reference book for anyone wishing to understand homoeopathy. The book covers a variety of topics of general interest which offer a deeper understanding and a more challenging awareness of homoeopathy, its indications, potential and scope of action.

The Principles, Art and Practice of Homoeopathy (£6.95)

A book which explains in simple language the principles of homoeopathic practice and prescribing. It includes chapters on :- Dosage, Potency, First and Second Prescriptions, Homoeopathic History Taking and The Consultation. A second section is concerned with Constitutional Prescribing and the role of homoeopathy in the treatment of Cancer.

Please send a s.a.e. for list of other available titles.